MW00900247

Medical Cannabis
For Chronic Pain Relief

American Veterans
For Cannabis Therapy

Author

Steven Leonard-Johnson, RN, PhD

DEDICATION

This Book Is Dedicated To All

United States Veterans

It is our hope that the information in this book will encourage more cannabis studies by the VA.

HOPE FOR VETERANS® PROGRAM

Community Hope Administrative Office

959 Route 46 East, Suite 402

Parsippany, NJ 07054

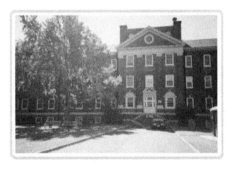

Hope for Veterans Transitional Housing Program, located at the VA New Jersey Healthcare Campus in Lyons NJ, has helped more than 430 veterans overcome homelessness and despair since 2004.

50% of the proceeds of this book will be donated to

The Hope for Veterans Program

to help further their cause.

Table of Contents

ACKNOWLEDGEMENTS

In memory of my father, Donald J. Leonard, a U.S. Navy Veteran (WW II), to my mother Elizabeth, and to my siblings Betty, Grace, and Donny.

A special thanks to Louis Manzo and Stacia McDonough, two of the very finest people, for their encouragement and support to me, and for their selfless dedication to our veterans. Mrs. Stacia McDonough is the widow/Gold Star Wife of highly decorated Vietnam veteran John E. McDonough, Sergeant U.S. Air Force.

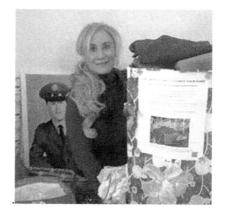

Photo Credit: Louis Manzo

Vietnam War
John E. McDonough, Sergeant U.S. Air Force
(pictured in flight suit on front cover)

This photograph was taken during her preparations for her 4th annual, "They Kept Us Safe, Let's Keep Them Warm," new clothing drive benefiting New Jersey's homeless veterans. Stacia McDonough is the founder of this now tremendously successful event. She is also a Member of the prestigious Hope for Veterans Leadership Committee, a NJ non-profit organization which houses formerly homeless veterans, and a proud member of Rolling Thunder, Inc.

I would like to give a special thanks to veterans Mary Lynn Mathre, RN, MSN, Co-founder and President of Patients Out of Time and founding member of the American Cannabis Nurses Association, and also to Al Byrne, LCDR, SC, USN ret., Co-Founder & Director Emeritus of Patients Out of Time and founding member of Veterans for Medical Cannabis Access. These veterans are the earliest pioneers and advocates that I know of in the country promoting cannabis for veterans. They have been advocating cannabis for veterans for several decades now.

Thanks to Dr. Ed Lueddeke, DC (chiropractic physician) and his wife Patty for their many years of friendship and help in seeing patients at my office, Acadia Advanced Therapy in Bar Harbor, Maine, and for exploring the metaphysical and energetic aspects of health. The Lueddeke's are the most well versed people I've ever known in the fields of metaphysics and health care.

Thanks to my dear and supportive friends Doug and Evangeline Wollmar and to Evangeline's dad, my dear friend Judge Charles Lincoln, may he rest in peace. Charles was a descendant of President Lincoln. He was lean and tall with great wit.

And to my dear friend and colleague Dr. Jay Goldman, DMD, MSW, chronic pain specialist and therapist extraordinaire, for all of his input and advice over the past few years. Of special note is the fact that Dr. Goldman has volunteered hundreds of hours of services to our veterans.

Also thanks to my longtime friends Ellen and Homer Ray and family of Nantucket, Massachusetts.

Lastly, I would like to thank Kelly Walker for her encouragement and support; otherwise this book would not have been possible.

Preface

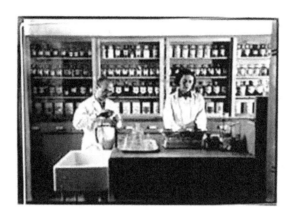

In order to fully understand the mechanism of action of cannabis, it will be necessary to give an overview of a recently discovered system in the body called the **endocannabinoid system (eCS)**. This is a system most professionals have never heard of, as we were never taught about the eCS in our formal education.

The eCS is a key regulator of homeostasis in vertebrates (having a spine) dating back 600 million years. However, due to the eCS being a relatively new discovery (1992), this information has not yet reached the professional classroom.

(There is generally a ten to thirty-year lag from the time of scientific discovery to the time it reaches the classroom. The discovery of the endocannabinoid system is a prime example of this delay in dissemination of information.)

Make no mistake about it; the discovery of the eCS system is one of the most important medical discoveries of our time.

In order to understand how medical cannabis works in your body, you will need to understand the endocannabinoid system and how it works.

This book will provide you with the basic information you will need in order to be more comfortable when working in cannabis therapeutics. At the rate medical cannabis is being accepted, used, and recommended, in a few years, most health professionals will be working with medical cannabis to some degree. The numbers of people being treated with cannabis are growing by the millions across the United States.

It is no secret that treating patients with medical cannabis remains a misunderstood and controversial topic to many. A new word has been coined in the cannabis industry for those who still fear using cannabis: *cannaphobia*. Contributing to the subset of cannaphobia, professional cannaphobia, are the wide ranges of laws concerning medical cannabis. The laws seem disorganized, ambiguous, and confusing, not only from state to state, but from state to federal level as well.

In Florida, during the last quarter of the year 2017, there were approx. 1250 doctors certified in cannabis medicine. 10% (125) of those doctors actually practiced cannabis medicine and 25% of them never renewed their cannabis certifications for 2018. Florida has approximately 50,000 doctors and 1/3 of them are over 60 years of age. For the most part cannabis medicine has not been taught in our nursing and medical schools and only a handful of schools are teaching about it now.

Another reason for slow assimilation of cannabis medicine in is that many practitioners feel they may face trouble from the authorities if they recommend cannabis.

Books like this attempt to fill the gaps of such rapid change in the world of medicine. Cannabis medicine is evolving so fast, that medical and nursing schools can't keep up with it, especially in cannabis prohibition states.

The purpose of writing this book was to keep people current in this new field of medicine, cannabis therapeutics.

REFERENCES

GW Pharmaceuticals. 2014. "GW Pharmaceuticals Announces that Sativex Receives Fast Track Designation from FDA in Cancer Pain." Last modified April 28. http://www.gwpharm.com/GW%20Pharmaceuticals%20Announc es%20that%20Sativex%20Receives%20Fast%20Track%20Designati on%20from%20FDA%20in%20Cancer%20Pain.aspx.

Savage, Sedden R., Kenneth L. Kirsh, and Steven D. Passik. 2008. "Challenges in Using Opioids to Treat Pain in Persons with Substance Use Disorders." *Addiction Science & Clinical Practice* 4(2): 4–25. http://www.ncbi.nlm.nih.gov/pmc/articles/PMC2797112/.

Disclaimer

Please note that the information in this book is for educational purposes only and is not meant as an alternative to medical diagnosis or treatment. The author makes no representations or warranties in relation to the health information in this book. If you think you may be suffering from any medical condition, you should seek medical attention. You should never delay seeking medical advice, disregard medical advice, or discontinue medical treatment because of information in this book. If you are considering making any changes to your lifestyle, diet, or nutrition, you should consult with your doctor.

These statements have not been evaluated by the Food and Drug Administration (FDA).

This information is not intended to diagnose, treat, cure, or prevent any disease.

FOREWORD

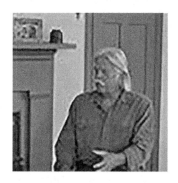

Al Byrne, LCDR, USN, ret.

Pain is best understood by recognizing that the severity of pain is what the patient says it is. Relief from pain carries the same definition and source.

Pain is not what the lawyers, judges, and law enforcement classes say it is. It is these three occupations that have dominated the treatment modalities for pain offered legally in the United States since 1941, 75 years. Worse, the medical class of the U.S. has abdicated their responsibility to this triad, not better informed than a gaggle of witches.

I am not a health care professional, nor do I have expertise in law or the judicial system. I am a DEA certified "cannabis expert." I have, with others, over the past three decades been dedicated to educating medical doctors, registered nurses, pharmacists, and scientists about the therapeutic value of the cannabis plant, and its interface with the Endocannabinoid System (ECS). I have done this by cobbling together worldwide science into a formal, accredited educational forum I co-founded+ named Patients Out of Time (www.medicalcannabis.com).

Concerning cannabis, the effort has been successful. I now believe that the "war on drugs", a misnomer - since inception the process has been a pogrom of hostility, and mendacity directed at citizenry marginalized by their race, sexual preference, or political stance - is in effect a "war on certain people." This failed war is about over.

About over is close but not a done deal. Patients, out of time, still die waiting for the United States to allow the herb cannabis to be reinstated into the US pharmacopoeia. A lot of them are Veterans.

Nine years ago a cohort* and I saw a need within the complex of myth and greed that fuels Americas prisons and courts to activate the same style of educational program that has brought 27 countries, 27 US states, Guam, The US Virgin Islands, DC and the Veterans Health Administration (VHA) to the understanding that the cannabis plant may be effectively used as a medicine.

In these nine years passed, knowledge of cannabis use for a multitude of physiological and emotional symptoms by military Veterans, of all countries, is now well known. Veterans for Medical Cannabis Access, which I co-founded, started the education process by continual, polite probing of the bureaucracy and thereby educating the leadership of the VHA. After three years in July of 2010, by official directive, the VHA declared the cannabis plant medicine and allowed its therapeutic use by any Vet living in and compliant with their states cannabis law. Overnight tens of thousands of US military Veterans had an alternative to the mind numbing, constipating opiates, and pharmaceuticals shoveled out by VHA personnel.

The VHA leadership, my partner and I, had done what we could at that time. It may seem to the reader that we all did well, that we should be proud of that huge change in US federal policy. I am, we are, but we also helped to create the most illogical, immoral, and medically unethical treatment modality in the history of modern medicine. I call it "medical treatment by geography" and its staggering inequality is being inflicted on United States of America's wounded Veterans!

In the VHA system patients are not equal. I live in Florida, and if I were to go to a VHA facility for care, admitting to cannabis use for my pain, security will be called and I will be escorted from the grounds and told not to return with cannabis in my system. If I checked in to a VHA clinic in Maine, I would be welcomed and thanked for my service to my country. This sucks!

It is reported that in our country 22 Veterans a day die by their own hand. Pain in all its meanings is suicide's agent. This is a minimum figure based on incomplete reporting from half the states. The real number hits around 50 a day, 18,250 lives lost each year. In Colorado where cannabis is legal for citizens 21 years of age and older the suicide rate immediately upon legalization dropped by 25 percent. A start and a statistical reality being replicated in other medical cannabis and recreational cannabis legal states.

A state with no positive cannabis law is led politically by a babbling array of compassion deprived ideologues. The cannabis laws that have been passed are insufficient, insure terrible medical outcomes, and are generally based on ignorance of the ECS and therapeutic applications. This is because the opponents and authors of such law are ignorant of the subject. That's bad, but what is awful and appalling is the ignorance of the medical and nursing community at large. There are 157 medical schools in the U.S. One, Temple University, teaches its students about the ECS and how the cannabis plant interacts with that system which is responsible for homeostasis in all living creatures excepting insects. Nursing schools scored zero. ECS knowledge is over twenty years old.

Our wounds and medical salvation are not recognized because of our zip code. A friend, Florida resident and combat Veteran of the Vietnam War asked me the question you should all ponder. Al, he said, "I went to Nam to fight for my country as I was asked, why now does my country not fight for me?

Another Brother, a 30 year Veteran of the Army, a retired Warrant Officer, skilled helicopter pilot, and nationally recognized air safety expert, made a case in front of a pile of North Carolina Senators that he and other Vets had found that cannabis helped them live a productive life and he and all of us should have the option to use cannabis medically. A lawyer, a Senator, ignorant as the rest chided my friend asking why he should believe and support the Vets. "Because I said so" was his answer. "I am a commissioned officer of the United States, as an officer, a leader; my word is all I have." The pilot stated the obvious and stood tall as he should. Has he and we not earned our right to equal medical treatment?

If not us then the rest of you are doomed to the feckless, foolish, dumb grapple of a cabal of cops and lawyers making medical decisions for me, my brothers and sisters - and you. Are "they" practicing medicine without a license?

My pain is physical: back, wrists, knee, and also emotional. I have been diagnosed with Post Traumatic Stress Syndrome, and my physical pain, is obvious to all who know me. I use cannabis every day to help me alleviate the physical pain and to keep me alive. That is true because I say so.

The words that follow mine will elaborate about the science, clinical experience, the applications, and various modalities explaining how the plant may be used for pain for a healthy life.

My words are placed here to inform you of an injustice to U.S. Veterans that can be rectified by the stroke of a President's pen, and a plant - cannabis.

Al Byrne, Lieutenant Commander, USN, ret.
Co-Founder & Director Emeritus of Patients Out of Time,
founding member of Veterans for Medical Cannabis Access.

June 2016, Franklin County Florida

+Mary Lynn Mathre, RN, MSN, CARN, Veteran
Co-founder and President of Patients Out of Time,
founding member of American Cannabis Nurses Association.

*Michael Krawitz, Sgt., USAF, ret.
Co-founder of Veterans for Medical Cannabis Access.

CHAPTER 1

A Brief History of Medical Cannabis as an Analgesic

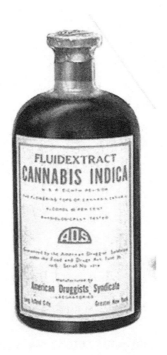

In the year 2737 BC, Chinese Emperor Shen-Nung wrote a book of treatment methods. In this book he wrote about using cannabis sativa for dozens of ailments. Cannabis Sativa is one of the 50 basic herbal medicines in traditional Chinese medicine (Drug Enforcement Administration Museum 2011 Sep; 27(9)).

Hua Tao (145–208 AD) was the first doctor in China not only to use anesthesia, but to use cannabis as an anesthetic. He concocted a brew called the cannabis boiling powder. It was used in surgery and consisted of herbs and wine mixed with cannabis to produce a pain-killing hallucinogenic tea. It was used in surgery of the head and abdomen (Drug Enforcement Administration Museum 2011 Sep; 27 (9)).

In *United States Pharmacopeia 1850–1941*, marijuana and hashish extracts were listed as the first, second, or third most prescribed medications in the United States from 1842 to the 1890s (Kowal 2015).

Major pharmaceutical companies such as Squibb, Eli Lily, and Parke Davis used cannabis in their formulas from 1854 to 1941. During these years, there were more than two thousand different pharmaceutical medications containing cannabis. These cannabis medicines, which addressed such ailments as anxiety, gout, insomnia, pain, and inflammation, were sold throughout the United States.

Chapter 1 References

[1] Drug Enforcement Administration Museum. "Cannabis, Coca, & Poppy: Nature's Addictive Plants".
https://www.deamuseum.org/ccp/cannabis/history.html

[2] Kowal, Andrew. 2015. "Opium, Marijuana, Oh My!" 2015
http://www.massmed.org/Continuing-Education-and-Events/Conference-Proceeding-Archive/Kowal-Handout/

CHAPTER 2

A Brief History of American Cannabis Prohibition

In 1936 the film *Reefer Madness* was introduced to the American public. This propaganda film was based on fiction; unfortunately, at the time an unsophisticated public took the film seriously. The purpose and design of this movie was to set the stage for cannabis prohibition. One year after this movie was released, the Marijuana Tax Act was introduced. This act restricted possession of marijuana for medical and industrial use. Those able to obtain cannabis incurred an excise tax for the privilege (Bestrashniy and Winters 2015).

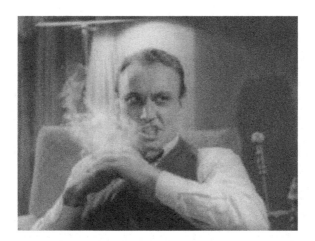

The Boggs Act of 1952 increased existing drug possession penalties fourfold. The Daniels Act of 1956 increased the penalties of the Boggs Act eightfold. The Narcotics Control Act of 1957 set mandatory sentencing for drug-related crimes, which included growing, possession, and distribution of marijuana. With this new law in place, a first marijuana offense carried the penalty of a minimum of two to ten years' imprisonment and a fine of up to $20,000 (Bestrashniy and Winters 2015).

A Schedule I drug is defined as one having "no medicinal value" and is considered only as being "hazardous to one's health." It is interesting to note that a National Institutes of Health report states that "THC has twenty times the anti-inflammatory potency of aspirin and twice that of hydrocortisone."

There has never been a recorded lethal dose of cannabis. It is no secret that cannabis has medicinal value, and cannabis is generally safe, especially when used responsibly under medical supervision. Clearly, cannabis is not in the same class as a Schedule I drug. However, cannabis was classified as a Schedule I drug in 1970, the handiwork of prohibitionists and others with much to gain from this bogus drug scheduling.

Skip ahead to the present. The latest law passed by the most recent act of Congress in February of 2016 is as follows: the federal government is now prohibited from raiding medical cannabis dispensaries in states where cannabis is legal. This new law is clearly a government stand-down on the war on drugs—at least on cannabis.

Research into cannabis as a medication is only in its infancy. US government grants to study cannabis are limited to $500,000, and researchers may only use smoked forms of cannabis. These parameters are small in scale compared to what pharmaceutical companies can spend.

Israel, in my opinion, is the most progressive country in the world when it comes to acceptance of cannabis and research. Currently, one of Israel's most publicized areas of cannabis research topics is on cannabis and bone healing. Researchers are finding out that cannabis greatly improves bone healing. Israel also uses cannabis in established settings, such as nursing homes and with the aged.

Israel's military has also allowed cannabis for the treatment of PTSD.

Chapter 2 References

[1] Bestrashniy, Jessica, and Kenneth C. Winters. 2015. "Variability in Medical Marijuana Laws in the United States." *Psychology of Addictive Behaviors: Journal of the Society of Psychologists in Addictive Behaviors* 29(3): 639–42.
http://www.ncbi.nlm.nih.gov/pmc/articles/PMC4588056/

[2] Manzanares, J., M. D. Julian, and A. Carrascosa. 2006. "Role of the Cannabinoid System in Pain Control and Therapeutic Implications for the Management of Acute and Chronic Pain Episodes." *Current Neuropharmacology* 4(3): 239–57.
http://www.ncbi.nlm.nih.gov/pmc/articles/PMC2430692/

[3] *Wikipedia*, s.v. "Medical Cannabis," 2015
https://en.wikipedia.org/wiki/Medical_cannabis#Pain

CHAPTER 3

Complications and Limitations of Opioid Treatment

Treatment of pain can be very challenging. There are always concerns of adverse effects, addiction, overdose, and risk versus benefits when prescribing pain medications. Pain is not always treated adequately with available opiates, antidepressants, and/or anticonvulsant drugs. For instance, if a person needs 10 milligrams of a pain medication, but he or she cannot take more than 5 milligrams due to their side effects, he or she will not be able to take enough opioid medication to alleviate all of their pain. This is only one example of many that challenge the clinician when trying to manage a patient's pain with opioids, whether the pain is chronic, intractable, cancer-associated pain, neuropathic, or central pain.

Opioids have a proven record and relative safety record alleviating acute pain and pain during terminal illness.

Opioids do not have proven efficacy or safety for treating chronic pain in the long term (Kowal 2015).

Ninety days is often used as a parameter for defining chronic pain. Studies show that after ninety days of continuous use, opioid treatment is more likely to become a lifelong need. Studies show that patients who continue opioids for more than ninety days tend to be high-risk patients (Kowal 2015).

A threshold of 100 milligrams per day daily total "morphine equivalent" is the key threshold. Daily morphine doses of more than 100 milligrams minimal effective dose (MED) are a red flag, as follows (Kowal 2015): In simple terms, when a person needs a high dose of painkiller to get minimal relief, they are at risk of an opioid overdose.

1.   Pain is not responsive.

2.   Insurmountable tolerance.

3.   Difficulty in controlling use.

4.   Misuse.

5.   Addiction.

6.   Diversion.

High Opioid Dose and Overdose Risk: On a scale of zero to twelve, number 4 below shows a threefold increase in opioid overdose risk when 100 milligrams per day of morphine equivalent is reached or exceeded (Benyamin et al. 2008).

1.   1 to 19 mg/day (1.00 on risk scale)

2.   20 to 50 mg/day (1.19 on risk scale)

3.   50 to 99 mg/day (3.11 on risk scale)

4.   <u>>100 mg/day **(11.18 on risk scale)**</u>

Side Effects: Finally, the role of opioids in the treatment of chronic pain is also influenced by the fact that these potent analgesics are associated with a significant number of side effects and complications.

Common side effects of opioid administration include the following:

- Sedation

- Dizziness

- Nausea/vomiting

- Constipation

- Physical dependence

- Tolerance

- Respiratory depression

Physical dependence and addiction are clinical concerns that may prevent proper dosing and in turn inadequate pain management.

Less common side effects of opioids may include the following (National Institute on Drug Abuse 2015):

- Delayed gastric emptying

- Hyperalgesia (increased sensitivity to pain)

- Immunologic and hormonal dysfunction

- Muscle rigidity myoclonus

The most common side effects of opioid usage are constipation (a very high incidence) and nausea. These two side effects can be difficult to manage. The side effects may be severe enough to require opioid discontinuation and contribute to under dosing and inadequate analgesia (pain relief).

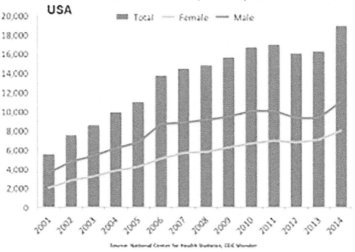

Number of Deaths from Prescription Opioid Pain Relievers USA

Source: National Center for Health Statistics, CDC Wonder

National Overdose Deaths

The figure above shows the total number of overdose deaths in the United States involving opioid pain relievers from 2001 to 2014.

The chart is overlaid by a line graph showing the number of deaths of females and males. From 2001 to 2014, the total number of deaths was a 3.4-fold increase (Bachhuber, Saloner, Cunningham, and Barry 2014).

Ten states (Alaska, Colorado, Hawaii, Maine, Michigan, Montana, Nevada, New Mexico, Rhode Island, and Vermont) enacted medical cannabis laws between 1999 and 2010. These states with medical cannabis laws had a 24.8 percent lower mean annual opioid overdose mortality rate compared with states without medical cannabis laws. (Benyamin et al. 2008). In simple terms, states with enacted medical cannabis laws had an average of 24.8% decrease in opioid deaths.

Chapter 3 References

[1] Bachhuber, Marcus A., Brendan Saloner, Chinazo O. Cunningham, and Colleen L. Barry. 2014. "Medical Cannabis Laws and Opioid Analgesic Overdose Mortality in the United States, 1999–2010." *JAMA Internal Medicine* 174(10): 1668–73.
http://archinte.jamanetwork.com/article.aspx?articleid=1898878&resultClick=3

[2] Benyamin, R., A. M. rescot, S. Datta, R. Buenaventura, R. Adlaka, N. Sehgal, S. E. Glaser, and R. Vallejo. 2008. "Opioid Complications and Side Effects." *Pain Physician*. 11(2 Suppl): S105–20.
http://www.ncbi.nlm.nih.gov/pubmed/18443635

[3] Kowal, Andrew. 2015. "Opium, Marijuana, Oh My!" 2015.
http://www.massmed.org/Continuing-Education-and-Events/Conference-Proceeding-Archive/Kowal-Handout/

[4] National Institute on Drug Abuse. 2015. "Overdose Death Rates." 2015
https://www.drugabuse.gov/related-topics/trends-statistics/overdose-death-rates

CHAPTER 4

Industrial Hemp Derived CBD

Industrial Hemp

Hemp cannot legally be grown in the United States unless government permission is granted. Large industrial hemp grows (up to 1200 acres) are being permitted around the United States at this time. CBD being sold over the counter in the United States has been derived from industrial hemp that has very low THC content and doesn't make a person high.

CBD can also be extracted from the marijuana sativa plants. These marijuana sativa plants can have much higher levels of THC than industrial hemp. Only CBD extracted from industrial hemp is being sold in cannabis prohibition states.

The two primary medicinal molecules (cannabinoids) in hemp and medical cannabis are:

1. **Delta-9-tetrahydrocannabinol (THC)** (a psychoactive molecule)

2. **Cannabidiol (CBD)** (a nonpsychoactive molecule)

These two molecules are very closely related in structure, as seen in these illustrations:

CBD (cannabidiol)

Cannabidiol (CBD)

THC (tetrahydrocannabinol)

US Government Patent #6,630,507:

"Cannabinoids as Antioxidants and Neuroprotectants"

Government studies have proven CBD to be a very safe and effective cannabinoid. A patent held by the US Department of Human Services, US Patent #6,630,507, October 7, 2003, states the following:

1. This patent recognizes CBD's ability as an antiepileptic, which means it is antiseizure.

2. CBD has powerful antioxidant activity that can be used in the prophylaxis (prevention) and treatment of oxidative associated diseases. Some of the conditions generally thought to be correlated with oxidative stress are Alzheimer's disease, Parkinson's disease, cancer, and autism.

3. CBD has the ability to lower intraocular pressure in the treatment of glaucoma.

4. CBD is protective to the brain from ischemic damage (helping blood and oxygen flow).

5. CBD is a naturally occurring constituent, hence a cannabinoid of the hemp plant and according to US government patent #6,630,507, it supports the nutritional health of aging bodies.

6. CBD has an anxiolytic effect, which means antianxiety.

7. CBD has neuro-protective properties, which means it protects the cells of the nervous system, the brain, and nerves in the body.

8. CBD has the ability to protect against cellular damage.

9. CBD does not have toxicity issues or serious side effects in large acute doses.

No signs of toxicity or serious side effects have been observed following chronic administration of cannabidiol (CBD) to healthy volunteers (Cunha et al., Pharmacology 21: 175–85, 1980), even in large acute doses of 700 milligrams/day (Consroe et al., Pharmacol. Biochem. Behav. 40: 701–8, 1991).

> Caution: *This does not mean people should be taking high doses of CBD. With any cannabis product, it is always recommended to start at a very low dose and increase gradually; more about this later.*

In addition, CBD researchers are also collectively building strong evidence of the following (Leonard-Johnson and Rappaport 2014; US Drug Enforcement Agency):

1. CBD is anticancer.
2. CBD lowers blood pressure.
3. CBD promotes bone growth.
4. CBD is antibacterial.
5. CBD is anti-inflammatory.
6. CBD suppresses muscle spasm.
7. CBD reduces seizures.
8. CBD is antianxiety.
9. CBD is antioxidant.
10. CBD relieves pain.

11. CBD regulates blood sugar.

12. CBD reduces autoimmune response.

THC Cannabinoid
(Known as: Marijuana, Cannabis sativa, Medical Cannabis)

There are more than five hundred compounds in Cannabis sativa plants (also called: called marijuana, cannabis sativa, medical cannabis, [this is not industrial hemp]). Many feel that Cannabis sativa extracted medicine is of a much higher quality than extracts from industrial hemp. *My other book: CBD-Rich Hemp Oil: Cannabis Medicine is Back, explains these cannabis classifications in detail.*

An effective dosing and titration of cannabis can come down to trial and error. Some strains of the plant can be effective where others are not. Also the route of administration can play an important role as to the tolerance and effectiveness of cannabis. Some people may tolerate cannabis by mixing it in a food, such as brownies, when they otherwise could not tolerate smoking it due to a respiratory condition for example; more about this later.

There are 120 or so aromatic terpenoids in cannabis plants, which give cannabis its distinctive scent when burned. Many researchers are of the opinion that these terpenoids have a direct and synergistic therapeutic effect with the cannabinoids and other compounds of the plant. A whole plant compound will be treated more as a food by the body than will a synthetic compound and will metabolize differently as well. Therefore, there is a general consensus among prescribers and users that the synthetic forms of the cannabinoid molecule will not be as effective or as well tolerated as whole extracts from the cannabis plant itself (Leonard-Johnson and Rappaport 2014).

Current research of the cannabis plant by pharmaceutical companies, and others, will prove to be very sophisticated. Developing specific strains is one way to get the proper medication a person needs. Other ways will be by design, combining specific extracts known to have a cause and effect on the body.

Keep in mind that some cannabinoids in whole plant medicine can have an opposite of the desired outcome. More sophisticated formulas, leaving out the negative acting cannabinoids and terpenes are being researched and developed at this time.

Further research is being done way beyond what is mentioned here, having to do with enzymes that act on cannabinoid regulation and still other research is focusing on cannabinoid interaction with other compounds; again, more about this later.

Chapter 4 References

[1] Leonard-Johnson, Steven L., and Tina Rappaport. 2014. *CBD-Rich Hemp Oil: Cannabis Medicine Is Back*. Scotts Valley, CA: CreateSpace. https://www.amazon.com/CBD-Rich-Hemp-Oil-Cannabis-Medicine-ebook/dp/B00K8IH3D6?ie=UTF8&qid=1418600126&ref_=tmm_kin_swatch_0&sr=1-1-catcorr

[2] PR Newswire. 2014. "Hemp as a Bio-Fuel Is One Step Closer to Reality." May 1. 2014 http://www.prnewswire.com/news-releases/hemp-as-a-bio-fuel-is-one-step-closer-to-reality-257504411.html

[3] US Drug Enforcement Agency. "Drug Schedules." http://www.justice.gov/dea/druginfo/ds.shtml

CHAPTER 5

The Basics of the Endocannabinoid System

The first cannabinoid was discovered in 1964 by Raphael Mechoulam, PhD. Dr. Mechoulam was a professor of medicinal chemistry and natural products at Hebrew University in Jerusalem, Israel. He was the first to synthesize the cannabinoid tetrahydrocannabinol (THC) (Leonard-Johnson and Rappaport 2014).

Three decades later, in 1992, Dr. Mechoulam made another important discovery. He and his team identified anandamide, a naturally occurring human neurotransmitter. Anandamide comes from the Sanskrit word *ananda*, which means bliss or delight. Anandamide, also known as N-arachidonoylethanolamine or AEA, is an endogenous cannabinoid neurotransmitter. The discovery of the neurotransmitter anandamide led to the subsequent discovery of the endocannabinoid system (Leonard-Johnson and Rappaport 2014).

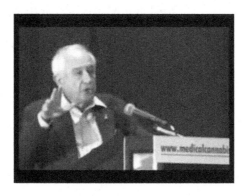

Raphael Mechoulam, PhD

Hence, in 1992, the newly discovered endocannabinoid system was named for the cannabis plant from which Dr. Mechoulam synthesized the first THC back in 1964. The endocannabinoid system is composed of receptor sites and endogenous endocannabinoids throughout the body. This widespread system is found in the brain, organs, glands, connective tissue, and immune cells, and it has regulatory roles in many physiological processes including appetite, pain sensation, mood, and memory. The primary purpose of this system revolves around maintaining homeostasis (Leonard-Johnson and Rappaport 2014).

The endocannabinoid system is an ancient, evolutionarily conserved, and ubiquitous lipid signaling system found in all vertebrates, which has important regulatory functions throughout the human body. The endocannabinoid system has been implicated in a very broad number of physiological as well as pathophysiological processes, including neural development, immune function, inflammation, appetite, metabolism and energy homeostasis, cardiovascular function, digestion, bone development, bone density, synaptic plasticity and learning, pain, reproduction, psychiatric disease, psychomotor behavior, memory, wake/sleep cycles, and regulation of stress and emotional states (Health Canada 2013).

The Five Major Functions
of the Endocannabinoid System

The endocannabinoid system is overall "silent"; however, it becomes transiently active "on demand" to help with these primary ECS functions (Health Canada 2013):

1.   **RELAX**—Reduction of pain and anxiety, modulation of body temperature, hormone production, smooth muscle tone, and blood pressure.

2.   **SLEEP**—Inhibition of motor behavior and sedation.

3.   **FORGET**—Extinction of adverse memories.

4.   **PROTECT**—Both at the cellular and emotional levels.

5.   **EAT**—Appetite-producing and reward-reinforcing effects.

Cannabinoid Classifications

1. **ENDOCANNABINOIDS** (endogenous cannabinoids): These are cannabinoids that occur naturally in the body. The two primary cannabinoids made by the body are:

   (AE)   N-arachidonoylethanolamine   or "anandamide"

   (2-AG) 2-arachidonoylglycerol

2. **PHYTOCANNABINOIDS** (plant cannabinoids): Cannabinoids in plant form are called phytocannabinoids. They are derived from the cannabis plant from the leaves, flowers, stem, and seeds.

3　**SYNTHETIC**　(made　in　a　lab):　Non-botanical cannabinoids.

4. **PURIFIED** Naturally occurring cannabinoids purified from plant sources.

(McPartland, Guy, and di Minzo 2014)

Regardless of type, cannabinoids act as neuromodulators and help regulate every physiological system such as our nervous system, digestive system, reproductive system, immune system, endocrine system, and muscular system.

Cannabinoids are an essential component involved in keeping the body systems balanced and stable, maintaining homeostatic balance (Leonard-Johnson and Rappaport 2014).

Primary Cannabinoids

1.　　**THC** (delta-9-tetrahydrocannabinol): The primary psychoactive, mind-altering cannabinoid found in cannabis.

2.　　**CBD** (Cannabidiol): The primary nonpsychoactive cannabinoid found in cannabis.

Receptor Sites of the Endocannabinoid System (ECS)

The system consists of the cannabinoid 1 and 2 (CB_1 and CB_2) receptors, the CB receptor ligands N-arachidonoylethanolamine (i.e. anandamide or AEA), and 2-arachidonoylglycerol (2-AG), as well as the endocannabinoid-synthesizing and degrading enzymes fatty acid amide hydrolase (FAAH) and monoacylglycerol lipase (MAGL) (Leonard-Johnson and Rappaport 2014).

Cannabinoid receptor sites are found throughout the entire body, embedded in the membranes of the cells. They act as lock-and-key-like chemical receptors. The cannabinoids have signals to which the receptors respond. The receptors receive the cannabinoids. We are just now beginning to understand how widespread and important the ECS is to our functioning.

There are two primary receptor sites of mention when working with phytocannabinoids: cannabinoid receptors CB_1 and CB_2. These two receptor sites have been identified and are found in the nervous system as well as the peripheral tissues and organs. These were discovered in 2003.

In the past ten years, the endocannabinoid system has been shown to be involved in a growing number of physiological functions in both the organs and the central and peripheral nervous systems. Researchers are finding out that, by modulating the endocannabinoid system, a number of diseases and pathological conditions may be alleviated.

Conditions such as multiple sclerosis, cancer, stroke, obesity/metabolic syndrome, anxiety disorders, neuropathic pain, Huntington's disease, myocardial infarction, movement disorders, hypertension, glaucoma, seizure disorders, Parkinson's disease, and osteoporosis are a sampling of the diseases helped, and there are many more.

The **cannabinoid receptor type 1**, often abbreviated as CB_1, is a G protein–coupled cannabinoid receptor located primarily in the central and peripheral nervous system. It is activated by the endocannabinoid neurotransmitters anandamide and 2-arachidonoyl glyceride (2-AG); by plant cannabinoids, such as the compound THC, an active ingredient of the psychoactive drug cannabis; and by synthetic analogues of binol (Leonard-Johnson and Rappaport 2014).

CB_1 receptors are ten times more abundant in the brain than mu opioid receptors, the receptors that are activated by morphine.

Few CB_1 receptors are found in the cardiorespiratory area of the brainstem, making cannabinoids safe in regard to the possibility of ever taking a fatal overdose (Health Canada 2013).

Brain regions rich with CB_1 receptors:

Region	Function
Nigrostriatal	Movement
Cerebellum	Fine motor movements
Hippocampus	Learning and memory
Nucleus accumbens	Drug reinforcement
Cerebral cortex	Higher cognitive functions

Moderate levels	Region Function
Hypothalamus	Temperature regulation
Amygdala	Emotionality
Brain stem	Sleep and arousal, nausea
Spinal cord	Pain

The **cannabinoid receptor type 2**, abbreviated as **CB₂**, a G protein–coupled receptor from the cannabinoid receptor family that in humans is encoded by the *CNR2* gene. It is closely related to the cannabinoid receptor type 1, which is largely responsible for the efficacy of endocannabinoid-mediated presynaptic-inhibition, the psychoactive properties of tetrahydrocannabinol (THC), the active agent in MARIJUANA, and other phytocannabinoids (natural cannabinoids). The principal endogenous ligand for the CB₂ receptor is 2-arachidonoylglycerol (2-AG) (Health Canada 2013).

CB₂ receptors are found primarily in the immune system, gastrointestinal system, brain, and peripheral nervous system.

The CB₁ and CB₂ receptors have the job of helping to regulate hormone and neuro-hormone activity. The fundamental function of the CB₁ and CB₂ receptors is either to "up-regulate" or to "down-regulate" neurotransmitter activity. This regulation process will determine how other hormones and body systems are regulated in the body.

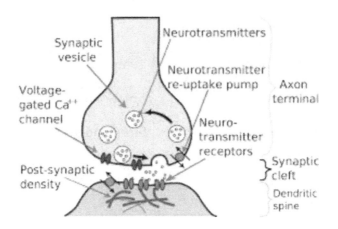

Typically, a nerve pathway travels in the direction from the presynaptic to the postsynaptic neuron, across the synaptic cleft. In contrast, retrograde nerve transmission of the ECS sends chemical signals in the opposite direction, from the postsynaptic to the presynaptic neuron, in order to regulate the presynaptic neurons production and release of neurotransmitters in response to the ECS retrograde feedback system.

The endocannabinoid system is a neuromodulatory system throughout the body, and it helps to keep the body in balance when exposed to endogenous and environmental insults. Consequently, it is easy to see how the minutiae of so many physiological systems may rely on the ECS. There is much yet to be learned about this system.

Endocannabinoids are produced on demand. They are often produced as an adaptive response to cellular stress and aimed at reestablishing cellular homeostasis. They are produced on demand in post synaptic neuronal cells and engage presynaptic CB receptors through this retrograde mechanism.

Endocannabinoids serve as topically active retrograde synaptic neurotransmitters. This means that they travel backward across the synaptic cleft from the postsynaptic to the presynaptic neurons, thereby providing feedback that directly up-regulates or down-regulates the release of other neuro-synaptic transmitters such as glutamate, dopamine norepinephrine and others.

Chapter 5 References

Health Canada. 2013. "Information for Health Care Professionals: Cannabis (Marihuana, Marijuana) and the Cannabinoids." 2013-06-12.
http://www.hc-sc.gc.ca/dhp-mps/marihuana/med/infoprof-eng.php

Leonard-Johnson, Steven L., and Tina Rappaport. 2014. *CBD-Rich Hemp Oil: Cannabis Medicine Is Back*. Scotts Valley, CA: Create Space.
https://www.amazon.com/CBD-Rich-Hemp-Oil-Cannabis-Medicine-ebook/dp/B00K8IH3D6?ie=UTF8&qid=1418600126&ref_=tmm_kin_s watch_0&sr=1-1-catcorr

McPartland, John, Geoffrey W. Guy, and Vincenzo di Minzo. 2014. "Care and Feeding of the Endocannabinoid System: A Systematic Review of Potential Clinical Interventions That Upregulate the Endocannabinoid System." *PLOS One* 9(3) e89566.
http://www.ncbi.nlm.nih.gov/pmc/articles/PMC3951193/

CHAPTER 6

Neuro Biological Aspects of
Medicinal Cannabis and Chronic Pain

My clinical background has been rounded out from more than thirty years of hospital-based nursing and working as a medical massage therapist and biofeedback therapist in the clinical office setting. I was first licensed as a massage therapist in 1980 and then graduated nursing school in 1985. I received my biofeedback and psychiatric nursing certifications in 1989. During my thirty-plus years as a massage therapist, I have easily performed thousands of medical massage therapy and clinical biofeedback sessions. I did not mention in my bio that I also did medical massage therapy out of Dr. Jhaveri's medical office in Middletown, New York. It was when working with Dr. Jhaveri that I received my most intensive training in the psychophysiological aspects of stress and pain management.

Also, in the summer of 1985, I was a massage therapist at Grossinger's Resort and Country Club in the Catskill Mountains in New York. I received a lot of invaluable training there from Grossinger's longtime resident masseur, a French physical therapist named Jules Bonnefin, PT, MsT. It was in the day-to-day work, apprenticing with the masters such as Jules and Dr. Jhavari, that I learned my trade.

Massage therapists tune into muscles, and muscles at the basic level are either "tight" or "relaxed." I was also able to see, by using EMG biofeedback, that people with tense muscles also showed signs of internalized systemic stress on the biofeedback monitors. The systemic stress however was expected, as we were working with people in treatment for anxiety and pain.

We knew stress and the symptoms of stress, anxiety, muscle tension especially, would cause increased levels of pain. We knew that muscle tension alone could cause pain. Muscle tension is usually caused by worrisome thoughts, fear, and surely from pain. Perseveration of negative thoughts can cause chronic stimulation of the sympathetic nervous system (fight or flight); consequently, they can cause or add to the symptoms of a chronic stress response.

Pain is stressful, and the body reacts by tensing muscle around that pain. Tensing one's muscles is usually an unconscious and habitual response to pain, which only makes the pain cycle worse. It can become an unconscious response. Nonetheless, this contraction response stresses the body even further. Biofeedback therapy is designed to help the patient become aware of his or her internalized tension, expressed in symptoms of the stress response, so he or she can get in tune with another opposite mechanism called the relaxation response.

Muscle tension further compounds the pain cycle by restricting blood flow to the tense and painful area. This in turn restricts oxygen and nutrients to the area to keep the tissue healthy.

This further compounds the problem by preventing metabolic waste from leaving the affected area. When lactic acid and other irritating metabolic waste build up due to lack of blood flow, the irritation from the metabolic acid waste causes what is called muscular "trigger points."

When I had my own office in Bar Harbor Maine, I worked with a chiropractor, Ed Lueddeke, DC, for many years. Dr. Lueddeke, an expert in muscular pain metabolism, taught me much about the subject. At one point we even incorporated a flotation tank to use in pain management, in which eight hundred pounds of medical grade Epsom salt was used to float people in a suspended gravity-like state. In this weightless state, people could let go of their muscle tension and learn to relax their tense areas, thereby helping to relieve their pain. By using medical massage therapy, biofeedback, chiropractic, and the float tank, we were able to get some very good results in pain reduction for our clients.

We were progressive back in the day, and we knew a lot about how to help people therapeutically. What we did not know about, however, was the endocannabinoid system, as it had not been discovered yet. Had we known about the endocannabinoid system and its role on the influence of pain and how it responds to stress, we would have seen our way more clearly. The ECS is a major regulation system in the body. We now know the ECS responds to stress in the defense of the body. The ECS system itself can also break down under too much stress. When our systems designed to respond to stress succumb to stress, that's when we know that we really have a problem.

The Autonomic Nervous System and

Physiological Stress in Pain Management

The stress response is an autonomic nervous system response, a "sympathetic" response. The relaxation response is also an autonomic nervous system response, a "parasympathetic" response. The sympathetic stress response, when it fires, puts demands and stress on our systems. It uses up more raw materials and fuels, such as vitamins, minerals, and hormones. All systems of the body will suffer from prolonged stress, which leads to depletions—not only physiological depletions, but depletions of emotions, mind, and spirit. Pain is stressful and easily can wear us out. The endocannabinoid system can be depleted or compromised under stress.

Chemical exposures to pesticides and environmental toxins can also compromise the ECS and the body's ability to produce neurohormones. When nutritional stress or environmental, emotional, and other leading causes of stress deplete us, this depletion can also lead to a condition now known as "Endocannabinoid Deficiency Syndrome" or "Clinical Endocannabinoid Deficiency."

The symptoms of "endocannabinoid deficiency syndrome" theory include: migraine headaches, fibromyalgia, and irritable bowel.

We've known about the body's systems and how these systems harmoniously work together for years. Now, the endocannabinoid system, no less important than any other body system, is the new kid on the block.

We need to see how the ECS will coexist with the other body systems. The nervous system is responsible for pain, no doubt, but the endocannabinoid system is responsible for the nervous system. Maybe this is why so many people get pain relief from cannabis. It regulates neurotransmission, and neurotransmission is how we experience pain.

Medications that help mood, especially the SSRI class of antidepressants, inhibit reuptake of serotonin, in order to leave more for use if there was ever a shortage, in theory. The endocannabinoid system, when functioning properly, will stimulate the presynaptic neuron to make more serotonin and tell the presynaptic neuron how much to fire. So how will the ECS impact psychiatry?

I am not anti-medication; I am pro-medication, when appropriate. I am realistic and have been in too many intense situations to know that psychiatric medications are essential, especially in acute care situations. There were times my knees were shaking in some acute care situations when I worked in the psychiatric emergency room at St Francis Hospital in Poughkeepsie, New York and at the state psychiatric facility in Bangor, Maine. When facing the possibility of severe assault by a psychotic person, psychotic secondary to an illegal drug reaction perhaps, then yes, you thank God for emergency medications and psychiatric stabilization medications to follow. It can be very dangerous work.

The point I am trying to make here is that each different system of the body, when depleted or compromised, needs to be treated with specific medications. Now, with the discovery of the endocannabinoid system, we need to realize that this system has its own specific medication, which is cannabis.

It either seems that some pain is relieved by treating the endocannabinoid system with cannabis alone, and this is enough, or maybe cannabis doesn't work at all, which is a clear indication that the pain is not going to be relieved by cannabis and the endocannabinoid system and the pain may not be originating from ECS influence.

In other cases, it seems that multiple systems need to be treated to relieve pain, including the muscle system, the nervous system (opioid system), and the endocannabinoid system. A properly regulated endocannabinoid system that is regulating the nervous system adequately, even in pain and aided by cannabis, can only be helpful. Other systems, such as the immune system, can come into play, causing inflammation secondary to an infection, and the inflammation is surely painful. As stated in the beginning of this book, a National Institutes of Health report states that THC has twenty times the anti-inflammatory potency of aspirin and twice that of hydrocortisone. Also mentioned is the potent anti-inflammatory property of CBD. In addition, CBD has antianxiety and antidepressive effects and suppresses muscle spasms.

Anxiety and depression can sometimes greatly negatively impact pain perception, and CBD helps to reduce these. These are the properties we know about in cannabis. There is much left to be explored. Cannabis has hundreds of compounds, terpenes, and bioflavonoids that so far have had very little study into their primary and synergistic combinations. We have only scratched the surface in cannabis research. What we do know, however, is that THC and CBD are a dream team of cannabinoids that have excellent pain reducing properties for many people; this is clear.

Hypothalamic-Pituitary-Adrenal Axis
(HPA Axis) in Stress Response

Our bodies have an "automatic" nervous system called the autonomic nervous system. It has two parts, one part that excites and stimulates us into defensive action (sympathetic nervous system) and the other part that stimulates relaxation (parasympathetic nervous system). These two opposing systems are designed to keep our automatic nervous systems in balance. The peak response of a sympathetic stress response is to fight or run. The peak response of the parasympathetic relaxation response is an orgasm. These two responses are polar opposite response systems of the autonomic nervous system and are the extremes of this automatic system.

In our society it is the stress response system that is most often triggered and in some cases chronically triggered. Our bodies need a balance between the stress response and the relaxation response to stay in balance and healthy. The stress system can become a chronic and dominant system, and when this happens, we are vulnerable to stress-related illness. Stressors that trigger the sympathetic system include pain, fear, heat, cold, emotional stress, imminent danger, toxic reactions, and just about any stimulus that can be stressful and noxious.

The stress response will shut down some body systems and stimulate others. The body systems the autonomic nervous system shuts down are the systems that are not needed in "fight or flight" stress response, such as the digestive system. The body systems that are ramped up are the systems the body needs to defend itself, such as the muscular system. It takes a lot of energy resources of the body to ramp up into the fight or flight mode.

The Stress Response

Body systems needed for defense are ramped up as follows:

1.   **HEART RATE** will increase.

2.   **RESPIRATION** will increase.

3.   **BLOOD VESSELS** will constrict to mitigate peripheral, if bleeding. When under attack, blood vessels will constrict in some parts of the body where they are not vital and will dilate in muscles where needed.

4.   **MUSCULAR SYSTEM** will tense for action.

5.   **BLOOD SUGAR** will increase for energy demands.

6.   **BLOOD CLOTTING** will speed up, in case of blood loss.

7.   **BLOOD PRESSURE** will increase.

8.   **VISION** will become tunnel vision.

9.   **EMOTIONS** such as anxiety and aggression may increase to deal with an attacker.

Systems not needed for defense are toned down as follows:

1.   **DIGESTION** will slow down.

2.   **AUDITORY** system will decrease hearing.

3.   **SEXUAL** system will inhibit erection.

4.   **BLADDER** can release contents.

The stress system is an adaptive system, meaning that if the stressors are not removed, we can adapt to them and stay chronically stressed. If the stress increases, we can adapt to that, too. In fact we can adapt right up until we reach the exhaustion phase, but after this phase is reached, it's downhill from there. If stress is prolonged and severe enough, death can occur.

The General Adaptation Syndrome theory was published by Hans Selye in 1936. He described it as follows:

Stress Exposure Triggered the Following Cycle

1.   **ALARM REACTION** activates the stress response.

2.   **RESISTANCE STAGE** is a stage in which the body will respond to stress until it is no longer needed and goes back to recovery and restoration or will be repeatedly stimulated, leading to the next phase.

3.   **EXHAUSTION PHASE** is the stage in which adaptive capability is burned out, and the stress-related adrenal glands become exhausted. This stage exposes the hippocampus area of the brain (emotion, memory), which becomes impaired and exposes the individual to anxiety and depression states. This stage makes the individual vulnerable to stress-related illness (Manzanares, Julian, and Carrascosa 2006).

4.   **DEATH** is the end result if stress is severe and never ending.

Our most vulnerable systems can wear out first under chronic stress. If we hold our stress in the muscular system, we may experience muscular pain, trigger points, and rigidity. If we hold our stress in our gut, we can experience digestive dysfunction and pain and so on down the list.

The stress system is an adaptive system; however, it can also be overwhelmed by a traumatic event or circumstance. This can be a physical injury, a psychologically traumatic event, or both. When overwhelming trauma is experienced, it does not give an individual time to adapt. It becomes an immediate issue; however, the mind has the ability to block out a traumatic event and can set the event aside to be dealt with at a later and better time. Essentially, this is a "built-in" psychological protective mechanism referred to as a post-traumatic stress response. In a sense this is a healthy response in a survival scenario, such as combat; however, it can be very debilitating if it is severe and left untreated.

This stress-response system in the body is known as the (limbic)-hypothalamic-pituitary-adrenal (HPA) axis. The HPA axis is an on-**demand system. When we are exposed to stressors, such as danger and thre**at, the HPA system will spring into action.

Another on-demand system is the endocannabinoid system. These two systems (the endocannabinoid system and the autonomic nervous system) do not respond in the same way, and they have different functions and triggers.

The stress response is a fight or flight or get out of danger system, while the endocannabinoid system is designed to bring the body back into balance. Both systems are protective in nature, and each system plays a role in pain. These two systems no doubt interact with each other, and we will explore this further. It is a more complicated and less understood area of psychophysiology.

Basically, the stress response action starts in the emotional centers of the brain, the amygdala (emotions, survival instincts, and memory), hippocampus (emotions, memory, spatial navigation), and prefrontal cortex (executive functioning). When the amygdala perceives danger, it sends a distress signal to the hypothalamus (command center to the rest of the body) (H). The hypothalamus secretes corticotropin-releasing hormone (CRF) and vasopressin.

These two peptides in turn stimulate adrenocorticotropic hormone (ACTH) from the pituitary gland. The ACTH in turn stimulates glucocorticoids from the adrenal gland, primarily cortisol, which is released into the blood stream to initiate the physiological stress response. Glucocorticoids in turn act back on the hypothalamus and pituitary (to suppress CRH and ACTH production) in a negative feedback cycle.

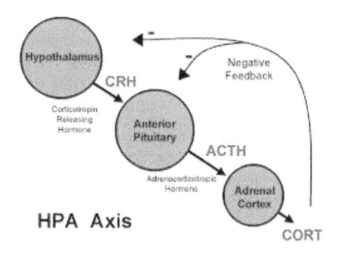

With repeated exposure to stress, the organism habituates to the stressor with repeated and sustained HPA axis activation. Therefore, it is important to support healthy cortisol levels in order to ensure that the hypothalamus and pituitary glands maintain the appropriate level of sensitivity to the negative feedback of cortisol.

Central secretion of phase I alarm chemicals, such as epinephrine and norepinephrine, as well as HPA axis activation and secretion of CRF, ACTH, and cortisol persist. Interestingly, with aging the hypothalamus and pituitary are less sensitive to negative feedback from cortisol, and both ACTH and cortisol levels rise as we age. Older women secrete more cortisol in response to stress than do older men. Young women, however, produce lower levels of cortisol in response to stress than do young men (Lise Alschuler, ND) 2014.

A chronic stress response can surely induce and promote continued pain. In the next section of this chapter, we will explore further how a chronic stress response can also affect the endocannabinoid system and pain management.

The Bio-Neurological Aspects of the

Endocannabinoid System in Chronic Pain

The endocannabinoid system has been recognized as a major neuromodulatory system, which functions to maintain brain homoeostasis (brain balance). Endocannabinoids are synthesized and released from the post synapse and act as retrograde neuronal messengers, which bind to cannabinoid type 1 receptors at the presynapse. Here, they inhibit the release of neurotransmitters, including glutamate and GABA. By these means, endocannabinoids control the activation of various neuronal circuits, including those involved in neuroendocrine stress processing.

When activated, the ECS will decrease stimulation to the stress response system through the retrograde feedback system. Accordingly, exogenous cannabinoids such as the major active component of marijuana, Delta (9)-tetrahydrocannabinol, have long been known to activate the major neuroendocrine stress response system (it will down-regulate the stress response) of mammals, the hypothalamic-pituitary-adrenocortical (HPA) axis (Steiner and Wotjak 2008).

Within the last decade, a large body of evidence has mounted indicating that the endocannabinoid system is involved in the central regulation of the stress response; however, the specific role endocannabinoid signaling plays in phases of HPA axis regulation and the neural sites of action mediating this regulation were not mapped out until recently (Steiner and Wotjak 2008).

Interestingly, there appears to be some anatomical specificity to the role of the endocannabinoid system in each phase of HPA axis regulation, as well as distinct roles of both anandamide and 2-arachidonoylglycerol in these phases. Overall, the current level of information indicates that endocannabinoid signaling acts to suppress HPA axis activity through concerted actions within the prefrontal cortex, amygdala, and hypothalamus.

Medical Cannabis in Pain Management as

Put Forth by the National Institutes of Health

Nociception is the "pain transmission system". These sensory receptors are spread throughout the body. When activated they send signals throughout the peripheral nervous system to the spinal cord and then travel to the brain. These signals are processed at each stage of transmission while traveling towards the brain via the peripheral and central nervous systems. The endocannabinoid system has CB1 receptors at these stages of transmission and when stimulated can have an influence on the modulation of the nociception signals (**pain transmission signals)** thereby down-regulating and modulating these pain signals.

Administration of natural or synthetic cannabinoid receptor agonists has shown therapeutic value for a number of important medical conditions, including pain (particularly against pain of neuropathic origin), anxiety, glaucoma, nausea, emesis, muscle spasms, and wasting diseases. Insofar as pain is concerned, it is well known that cannabinoid receptor agonists have antinociceptive and anti-hyperalgesic effects at the peripheral and central (spinal and supraspinal) levels, as has been demonstrated in acute and chronic pain models (Iverson and Chapman 2002; Pertwee 2001).

Cannabinoid receptors and endocannabinoids are present in pain circuits from the peripheral sensory nerve endings up to the brain. Cannabinoid receptor agonists modulate nociceptive thresholds by regulating neuronal activity (Hill and Tasker 2012), but they also relieve pain by acting on non-nervous tissues. (Small-Howard, Shimoda, Adra, and Turner 2005).

On the other hand, although CB_2 receptors have been related traditionally to the peripheral effects of cannabinoids (mainly modulation of the immunologic responses), they also contribute to anti-nociception (**lowering pain transmission signals)** by inhibiting the release of proinflammatory factors by non-neuronal cells located near nociceptive (**pain transmission signals)** neuron terminals. CB_2 receptors are expressed in several types of inflammatory cells and immunocompetent cells. For that reason, activation of peripheral CB_2 receptors generates an anti-nociceptive response (**lowering pain transmission signals)** in situations of inflammatory hyperalgesia (heightened pain perception) and neuropathic pain.

The biochemical mechanisms involved in the interaction between cannabinoid and opioid receptors relate to the transduction and release of diverse mediators involved in the modulation of nociception and inflammation. On the other hand, cannabinoid receptor agonists induce the synthesis and/or release of endogenous opioid peptides (Corchero, Avila, Fuentes, and Manzanares 1997; Manzanares et al. 1999). Sub chronic treatment with THC produces an increase in opioid gene expression in the spinal cord, sustaining the hypothesis of an interaction between the cannabinoid and opioid systems in this region.

Opioid Synergism

The combination of two antinociceptive drugs acting through specific receptor systems yields major benefits. When given in combination with synergistic substances, the required dose of each agent can be reduced to less than would be explained by a simple additive effect. The clinical benefit of this property is important in analgesic treatments, because effective pain relief can be achieved with fewer or no side effects.

The opioid system is one of the systems interacting with the cannabinoids that has been most explored (Corchero, Manzanares, and Fuentes 2004; Fuentes et al. 1999; Fuentes et al. 1999). Electrophysiological analysis of the effects of cannabinoids on RVM (rostral ventromedial medulla) has revealed that cannabinoids have effects similar to those elicited by morphine (Meng, Manning, Martin, and Fields 1998). Cannabinoid and opioid receptors both exist at various levels in the pain circuits, and these two systems may operate synergistically. THC and morphine have been shown to act synergistically, mutually potentiating their antinociceptive actions.

Cannabidiol (CBD) is another major constituent of the cannabis sativa plant, having the same therapeutic effects as THC (analgesic, anti-inflammatory, and others) but with a different pharmacologic profile. Studies have been made with cannabidiol derivatives developed to inhibit peripheral pain responses and inflammation after binding to cannabinoid receptors. Interestingly, some of these cannabidiol derivatives did not have central nervous system effects but maintained their antinociceptive and anti-inflammatory properties. This means that centrally inactive synthetic cannabidiol analogues may be good candidates for the development of analgesic and anti-inflammatory drugs for peripheral conditions (Fride et al. 2004).

Acute Pain

Opioids are powerful analgesics widely utilized in clinical pain management, but they yield a poor analgesic response in conditions of certain pathologic pain, such as neuropathy. THC induces antinociception in rats with pathologic pain after nerve injury. Moreover, THC antinociception is independent of opioid receptors in rats with some pathologic pain, as the antinociceptive effect after nerve injury is blocked by the CB_1 receptor antagonist SR141716A but not by the opioid receptor antagonist naloxone, and there is no cross-tolerance between the antinociceptive effects of morphine and THC (Mao et al. 2000). Therefore, THC and other cannabinoids may be superior to opioids in alleviating intractable pathologic pain syndromes.

Multiple Sclerosis

Multiple sclerosis (MS) is a lifelong chronic disease in which nerve cells are attacked by the immune system, originating painful muscle spasms and many other problems, including neuropathic pain. There are about 1.1 million sufferers of MS worldwide. Clinical trials have tested the potential medical applications of cannabis for the treatment of MS symptoms, although some of them present a small number of patients; there is also data from responses to questionnaires (Iversen 2003; Pertwee 2002). <u>Smoking cannabis not only has helped to stop spasms, but also has halted the progression of multiple sclerosis.</u>

Neuropathic Pain

Severe neuropathic pain has proved difficult to treat, and evidence suggests that none of the available drugs, mainly opioids, are effective in more than 50 percent of patients. This is an area of significant unmet clinical need.

It is important to emphasize that cannabinoid receptor agonists are more effective than opioids in the management of neuropathic pain. Different hypotheses have been proposed to explain this phenomenon (Mao et al. 2000). One is based on the presence of cannabinoid receptors in primary afferent myelinated A-fibers, since this pain is partly due to spontaneous discharge of these fibers (Hohmann and Herkenham 1999). The A-fibers contain fewer μ-opioid receptors than cannabinoid receptors. There is evidence confirming this hypothesis.

Cancer Pain

Pain is one of the most frequent symptoms in patients with cancer, and the World Health Organization recommends that they receive adequate pain relief. Cannabinoids are among the compounds under development for the treatment of these patients, and they seem to have analgesic activity (Radbruch and Elsner 2005).

Clinical trials are also underway to assess the effectiveness of cannabis extract preparations (containing THC and CBD) for the relief of cancer pain (neuropathic related cancer pain).

Fibromyalgia

This disease is characterized by the presence of generalized pain throughout the body, confirmed by the presence of tender and painful points on digital palpation in at least eleven of the eighteen points established for diagnosis. Pharmacologic treatment usually consists of tricyclic antidepressants combined with NSAIDs. Although there are no specific clinical studies of the use of cannabinoid receptor agonists for symptomatic relief of this disease, data that support their therapeutic potential, thanks to their anti-inflammatory and sedative properties (Russo 2004). Clinical endocannabinoid deficiency (CECD): Can this concept explain therapeutic benefits of cannabis in migraine, fibromyalgia, irritable bowel syndrome, and other treatment-resistant conditions?

Spasticity

Spasticity entails increased resistance to passive movement. Among other disadvantages, it causes pain per se and is also secondary to joint stiffness. Among the therapeutic measures proposed are the elimination or reduction of nociceptive stimuli, rehabilitation (occupational physical therapy), and the use of antispasmodic medication. Clinical trials have evaluated the efficacy of cannabinoids in diverse musculoskeletal entities accompanied by severe spasticity.

Conclusion

Clinical trials seem to indicate that either extracts of the cannabis sativa plant containing known amounts of the active compounds (mainly THC and CBD) or diverse synthetic derivatives of THC are promising treatments for painful conditions that do not respond to available treatments, such as neuropathic, inflammatory, and oncologic pain.

Specifically, cannabis extracts have shown effectiveness to relieve some symptoms in patients with multiple sclerosis, mainly for pain and spasticity. Pharmacologic manipulation directed to elevate endocannabinoids levels with, for example, anandamide reuptake inhibitors or by inhibiting the enzyme fatty acid amide hydrolase (FAAH), which is responsible for intracellular anandamide degradation, may well become a valuable therapeutic tool. CB_2 receptor selective agonists with no central effects are other promising pain treatments under investigation.

Pain severely impairs quality of life. Currently available treatments, generally opioids and anti-inflammatory drugs, are not always effective for certain painful conditions. The discovery of the cannabinoid receptors in the 1990s led to the characterization of the endogenous cannabinoid system in terms of its components and numerous basic physiologic functions. CB_1 receptors are present in nervous system areas involved in modulating nociception, and evidence supports the role of the endocannabinoids in pain modulation. Basic research on how cannabinoid receptors and endocannabinoids intervene in pain mechanisms is progressing rapidly. Clinical progress, however, is slow.

Cannabinoids have antinociceptive mechanisms different from those of other drugs currently in use, which opens a new line of promising treatments to mitigate pain that fails to respond to the pharmacologic treatments available, especially for neuropathic and inflammatory pain. The combination of cannabinoids with synergistic analgesic substances is interesting, because it may improve the efficacy and safety of treatment. One of the drawbacks of investigating cannabinoids is their typification as substances of abuse. However, compounds blunting severe pain allow patients to perform daily activities more easily, so the potential benefits should be weighed against possible adverse effects.

Our current understanding of the physiology and pharmacology of the endogenous cannabinoid system has motivated cannabis-based therapeutic drug design, in which attempts are being made to synthesize compounds with the desired therapeutic actions but without psychoactive adverse effects. Medications prepared with cannabinoid receptor agonists or with drugs that enhance endocannabinoid function (by either increasing release or diminishing reuptake of endocannabinoids) may afford the novel therapeutic approaches demanded by disorders in which pain is a prominent symptom.

Clinical trials seem to indicate that either extracts of the cannabis sativa plant containing known amounts of the active compounds (mainly THC and CBD) or diverse synthetic derivatives of THC are promising treatments for painful conditions that do not respond to available treatments, such as neuropathic, inflammatory, and oncologic pain. Specifically, cannabis extracts have shown effectiveness to relieve some symptoms of patients with multiple sclerosis, mainly for pain and spasticity (Manzanares, J., M. D. Julian, and A. Carrascosa 2006).

Chapter 6 References

[1] Corchero, J., M. A. Avila, J. A. Fuentes, and J. Manzanares. 1997. "Delta 9-Tetrahydrocannabinol Increases Prodynorphin and Proenkephalin Gene Expression in the Spinal Cord of the Rat." *Life Sciences* 61: L39–L43. http://www.ncbi.nlm.nih.gov/pubmed/9244374.

[2] Corchero J., J. Manzanares, and J. A. Fuentes. 2004. "Cannabinoid/Opioid Crosstalk in the Central Nervous System." *Critical Reviews in Neurobiology* 16: 159–72. http://www.ncbi.nlm.nih.gov/pubmed/15581411

[3] The Essence of Stress Relief. Year of Accessed/Last Modified Date Needed. "Hans Selye's General Adaptation Syndrome." http://www.essenceofstressrelief.com/general-adaptation-syndrome.html

[4] [Fride, E., C. Feigin, D. E. Ponde, A. Breuer, L. Hanus, N. Ar-shavsky, and R. Mechoulam R. 2004. "Cannabidiol Analogues Which Bind Cannabinoid Receptors but Exert Peripheral Activity Only." *European Journal of Pharmacology* 506: 179–88. http://www.ncbi.nlm.nih.gov/pubmed/15588739

[5] Fuentes, J. A., M. Ruiz-Gayo, J. Manzanares, G. Vela, I. Reche, and J. Corchero. 1999. "Cannabinoids as Potential New Analgesics." *Life Sciences* 65: 675–85. http://www.ncbi.nlm.nih.gov/pubmed/10462068

[6] Hill, M. N. and Tasker, J. G. 2012. "Endocannabinoid Signaling, Glucocorticoid-Mediated Negative Feedback, and Regulation of the Hypothalamic-Pituitary-Adrenal Axis." *Neuroscience* 204: 5–16. http://www.ncbi.nlm.nih.gov/pubmed/22214537

[7] Hohmann A. G., and M. Herkenham. 1999. "Localization of Central Cannabinoid CB1 Receptor Messenger RNA in Neuronal Subpopulations of Rat Dorsal Root Ganglia: A Double-Label *in situ* Hybridization Study. *Neuroscience* 90: 923–31. http://www.ncbi.nlm.nih.gov/pubmed/10218792

[8] Iversen, L. 2003. "Cannabis and the Brain." *Brain* 126: 1252–70.
http://www.ncbi.nlm.nih.gov/pubmed/12764049

[9] Iverson, L. and V. Chapman. 2002. "Cannabinoids; A Real Prospect for Pain Relief?" *Current Opinion in Pharmacology* 2(1): 50–55.
http://www.ncbi.nlm.nih.gov/pubmed/11786308

[10]Manzanares, J., J. Corchero, J. Romero, J. J. Fernandez-Ruiz, J. A. Ramos, and J. A. Fuentes. 1999. "Pharmacological and Biochemical Interactions between Opioids and Cannabinoids. *Trends in Pharmacological Sciences* 20: 287–94.
http://www.ncbi.nlm.nih.gov/pubmed/10390647

[11] Manzanares, J., M. D. Julian, and A. Carrascosa. 2006. "Role of the Cannabinoid System in Pain Control and Therapeutic Implications for the Management of Acute and Chronic Pain Episodes." *Current Neuropharmacology* 4(3): 239–57.
http://www.ncbi.nlm.nih.gov/pmc/articles/PMC2430692/

[12] Mao, J., D. D. Price, J. Lu, L. Keniston, and D. J. Mayer. 2000. "Two Distinctive Antinociceptive Systems in Rats with Pathological Pain. *Neuroscience Letters* 280: 13–16.
http://www.ncbi.nlm.nih.gov/pubmed/10696800

[13] Meng, I. D., B. H. Manning, W. J. Martin, and H. L. Fields. 1998. "An Analgesia Circuit Activated by Cannabinoids." *Nature* 395: 381–83.
http://www.ncbi.nlm.nih.gov/pubmed/9759727

[14] Pertwee, R. G. 2001. "Cannabinoid Receptors and Pain." *Progress in Neurobiology* 63: 569–611.
http://www.ncbi.nlm.nih.gov/pubmed/11164622

[15] Pertwee, R. G. 2002. "Cannabinoids and Multiple Sclerosis." *Pharmacology & Therapeutics* 95: 165–74.
http://www.ncbi.nlm.nih.gov/pubmed/12182963

[16] Radbruch, L. and F. Elsner. 2005. "Emerging Analgesics in Cancer Pain Management. *Expert Opinion on Emerging Drugs* 10: 151–71.
http://www.ncbi.nlm.nih.gov/pubmed/15757410

[17] Russo, E. B. 2004. "Clinical Endocannabinoid Deficiency (CECD): Can This Concept Explain Therapeutic Benefits of Cannabis in Migraine, Fibromyalgia, Irritable Bowel Syndrome and Other Treatment-Resistant Conditions?" *Neuroendocrinology Letters* 25: 31–39.
http://www.ncbi.nlm.nih.gov/pubmed/15159679

[18] Small-Howard, A. L., L. M. Shimoda, C. N. Adra, and H. Turner. 2005. "Anti-Inflammatory Potential of CB1-Mediated CAMP Elevation in Mast Cells." *Biochemical Journal* 388 (pt 2): 465–73.
http://www.ncbi.nlm.nih.gov/pubmed/15669919

[19] Steiner, M.A. and C. T. Wotjak. 2008. "Role of the Endocannabinoid System in Regulation of the Hypothalamic-Pituitary-Adrenocortical Axis." *Progress in Brain Research* 170: 397–432.
http://www.ncbi.nlm.nih.gov/pubmed/18655899

[19] Lise Alschuler, ND, 2/28/2014, Integrative Therapeutics, "The HPA Axis"
http://www.integrativepro.com/Resources/Integrative-Blog/2014/The-HPA-Axis

CHAPTER 7

FDA-Approved Synthetic Cannabinoid Medications Already in Use

Synthetic THC cannabinoids have been used in modern medicine since 1985. There are two synthetic THC cannabinoid medications approved by the FDA at this time, Marinol and Cesamet. These medications were approved by the FDA because they are "synthetic cannabinoids" and are not classified as Schedule I controlled narcotics. Natural plant cannabinoids that are derived from medical marijuana are still classified as Schedule I controlled substances. The Schedule I designation of the natural plant has created a block in research, as studies with Schedule I drugs are extremely difficult to get approval for in the United States.

The Two FDA-Approved

Synthetic THC Cannabinoid Medicines

Marinol (Dronabinol)

(Schedule III under US Controlled Substances Act)

Semisynthetic Delta-9 tetrahydrocannabinol (THC) was approved by the FDA in May of 1985 to help with anorexia associated with weight loss in patients with AIDS and for nausea and vomiting associated with cancer chemotherapy. Marinol can be used when conventional antiemetics have failed to help.

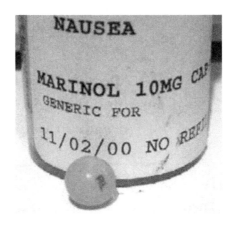

Standard dosage of Marinol is 2.5 milligrams to 10 milligrams twice a day. Patients prescribed Marinol frequently report that its psychoactive effects are far greater than those of natural cannabis. Patients report Marinol is more psychoactive than whole plant medicine. Marinol is not approved for use as an analgesic in the United States.

Cesamet (Nabilone capsule)

(Schedule II under US Controlled Substances Act)

Cesamet was approved by the FDA in 1985, withdrawn from the market in 1989, and then made available again in 2006. Cesamet is a synthetic cannabinoid for oral administration. Standard dosage is 1 milligram to 2 milligrams twice a day.

Chemically, Nabilone is similar to the active ingredient found in naturally occurring cannabis sativa L. (Marijuana; delta-9-tetrahydrocannabinol [delta-9-THC]).

Cesamet capsules are indicated for the treatment of the nausea and vomiting side effects associated with chemotherapy. Cesamet is used with patients who have failed to respond adequately to conventional antiemetic treatments. This restriction is required because a substantial proportion of any group of patients treated with Cesamet can be expected to experience disturbing psychotomimetic (symptoms similar to those of psychosis) reactions not observed with other antiemetic agents. Cesamet is used off-label to treat fibromyalgia pain.

Because of its potential to alter the mental state, Cesamet is intended for use under circumstances that permit close supervision of the patient by a responsible individual, particularly during initial use and dose adjustments.

Neither Marinol nor Cesamet is popular, due to their high cost, titration difficulties, dysphoric reactions, and the problem of the patient feeling intoxicated.

Chapter 7 References

[1] US Food and Drug Administration. 2004. "Marinol."
http://www.fda.gov/ohrms/dockets/dockets/05n0479/05N-0479-emc0004-04.pdf

[2] US National Library of Medicine. Updated 2007. "Cesamet—Nabilone Capsule."
https://dailymed.nlm.nih.gov/dailymed/drugInfo.cfm?setid=a7a2a4e1-9ecd-4e59-82b5-2068b5e50164

CHAPTER 8

The Two Current Pharmaceutical Plant-Based Cannabis Medications' Clinical Trials in the United States

Two pharmaceutical medications currently being studied in clinical trials in the United States are actual cannabis plant-based medications, not synthetic like Marinol and Cesamet. These plant-based medicines, Sativex and Epidiolex, were created by GW Pharmaceuticals, which has been in business since 1998. GW Pharmaceuticals distributes to many countries and <u>has had an estimated annual production of one hundred tons of medicinal cannabis since 2012 (GW Pharmaceuticals 2014)</u>.

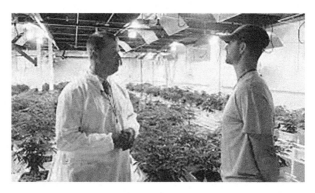

GW Pharmaceuticals: A cannabis-based pharmaceutical company.

Sativex (nabiximols)

In June of 2010, GW Pharmaceutical commercialized the world's first plant-derived cannabinoid prescription drug, Sativex, which is approved for the treatment of spasticity due to multiple sclerosis in twenty-five countries. Sativex is also in Phase 3 clinical development as a potential treatment of pain in people with advanced cancer. This Phase 3 program is intended to support the submission of a new drug application for Sativex in cancer pain with the US Food and Drug Administration and in other markets around the world (GW Pharmaceuticals 2014).

Each 100 microliter spray contains 2.7 milligrams delta-9-tetrahydrocannabinol (THC) and 2.5 milligrams cannabidiol (CBD), derived from cannabis sativa L. A patient may take up to sixteen sprays in a day (43.2 milligrams of THC and 40 milligrams of CBD daily total) of this botanical whole plant extract.

Sativex is indicated as treatment for symptom improvement in adult patients with moderate to severe spasticity due to multiple sclerosis (MS) who have not responded adequately to other antispasticity medication and who demonstrate clinically significant improvement in spasticity related symptoms during an initial trial of therapy (GW Pharmaceuticals 2014).

Epidiolex

Epidiolex is GW Pharmaceuticals' proprietary product candidate that contains a liquid formulation of highly purified plant-derived cannabidiol (CBD) as its active ingredient. Epidiolex is in development as a treatment for various orphan pediatric epilepsy syndromes. In 2015 Epidiolex was granted orphan drug designation by the FDA in the treatment of Dravet and Lennox-Gastaut syndromes, each of which is a severe infantile-onset, drug-resistant epilepsy syndrome. The FDA has granted expanded access INDs (investigational new drugs) to several independent investigators in the United States to allow treatment of pediatric epilepsy patients with Epidiolex (GW Pharmaceuticals 2014).

Of these four medications, Epidiolex is the only one that is THC free; however, it contains trace amount of other cannabinoids. It is a cannabidiol (CBD) only medication.

Chapter 8 References

[1] GW Pharmaceuticals. 2014. "Frequently Asked Questions." http://www.gwpharm.com/FAQ.aspx

[2] GW Pharmaceuticals. 2014. "GW Pharmaceuticals Announces that Sativex Receives Fast Track Designation from FDA in Cancer Pain." http://www.gwpharm.com/GW%20Pharmaceuticals%20Announces%20that%20Sativex%20Receives%20Fast%20Track%20Designation%20from%20FDA%20in%20Cancer%20Pain.aspx

CHAPTER 9

Medicinal Cannabis and Dentistry

Cannabis, commonly known as marijuana, is currently gaining an intense increase in use and popularity around the globe. Therefore, oral health care providers are likely to encounter patients who are regular users.

Cannabis "abusers" generally have poorer oral health than nonusers, with an increased risk of dental caries and periodontal diseases. Cannabis smoke acts as a carcinogen and is associated with dysplastic changes and premalignant lesions within the oral mucosa (a concept being challenged by recent cannabis research) (Cho, Hirsch, and Johnstone 2005).

Users are also prone to oral infections, possibly due to the immunosuppressive effects (a concept also being challenged by current cannabinoid research). Dental treatment of patients intoxicated on cannabis can result in the patient experiencing acute anxiety, dysphoria, and psychotic-like paranoiac thoughts. The use of local anesthetic containing epinephrine may seriously prolong tachycardia already induced by an acute dose of cannabis. Oral health care providers should be aware of the diverse adverse effects of cannabis on general and oral health and incorporate questions about patients' patterns of use in the medical history (Cho, Hirsch, and Johnstone 2005).

When dental professionals are aware of cannabis-smoking patients, they can use this information to assess whether or not the smoking of cannabis and the resulting "dry mouth" effect are causing adverse effects or initiating an active disease process, just as they would for heavy smokers.

Medical Cannabis-Assisted Dentistry

On the flip side of cannabis abuse and its negative effects on the oral mucosa and mental health, some dental practices are offering their patients medical cannabis as a way to reduce anxiety during a dental procedure. Medical cannabis-assisted dentistry is reported to be wildly popular in some areas of California. In fact, the state of California is considering dental anxiety as a qualifying condition for recommending medical cannabis in the area of sedation dentistry.

Given the positive effects cannabis can have, such as anxiety reduction, it is no wonder that cannabis has also found its way into the dental office. Of course the cannabis laws are different from state to state, and this treatment is a very limited option that is nonexistent in most states.

Hemp-Based Oral Care

Ironically, we would not expect to find hemp-based products in dentistry, especially after reviewing the mountain of literature linking smoked cannabis to oral disease, as pointed out previously.

However, it turns out that the protective properties of the cannabinoids in cannabis actually contain the very qualities needed to protect oral tissue and promote oral health. Cannabis contains more than one hundred cannabinoids; the two most well-known are THC and CBD. There are other cannabinoids in cannabis that are rarely mentioned; however, these also have very desirable protective properties. The cannabinoids used in these new dental products have exactly these desired qualities.

The Future of Dentistry

The future of dentistry may be based on the endocannabinoid system (ECS) and the cannabinoid-based products that are now being developed. Toothpaste, dentifrice, and mouthwash (gargling) have been around for centuries; this will not change, although perhaps the ingredients will (Nasdaq 2015).

Cannabinoids are known to have anti-inflammatory, antibacterial, anti-proliferative, and regenerating effects. Cannabinoids are also known to have anticancer qualities. There are already a few dental products in the marketplace that are cannabinoid based, and many others in research and development are cannabinoid based as well. Since the discovery of the endocannabinoid system in 1992 and the realization that the ECS is a built-in protection system of the body, it stands to reason that we can expect to see an explosion of cannabis-based products in the future.

Cannabinoid Research

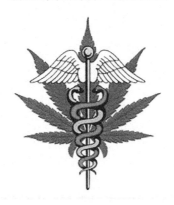

As we have discussed, some cannabinoids are legal in the United States, and some are not. THC is a Schedule I cannabinoid and obviously not legal, as it is psychoactive. We will not be seeing THC-based products in the general commercial marketplace. However, cannabidiol (CBD) is a nonpsychoactive cannabinoid and can be sold anywhere.

The nonpsychoactive CBD cannabinoid is totally legal in all fifty states (although it must be imported, as explained earlier) and in many countries around the world. CBD is being added to many products from shampoo to coffee, and there seems no end in sight to this trend. CBD is being added to food and cosmetics at a dizzying rate. It was only a matter of time before the dental industry picked up this trend.

Cannabinoids Helpful in Oral Care

The primary nonpsychoactive cannabinoids of interest in dentistry are CBD, CBG, CBGA, and CBCA. (There are dozens of other cannabinoids not yet fully researched at this time.)

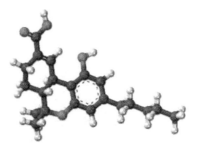

CBD

(Cannabidiol)

Antibacterial

Anti-inflammatory

Relieves pain

Anxiolytic

Antispasmodic

Antiseizure

Anticancer

Neuroprotectant

CBG

(Cannabigerol)

Aids sleep

Inhibits cancer cell growth

Promotes bone growth

Slows bacterial growth

CBGA

(Cannabigerolic acid)

Reduces inflammation

Relieves pain

Slows bacterial growth

CBCA

(Cannabichrome carboxylic acid)

Reduces inflammation

Treats fungus infection

The following cannabinoids have similar oral health properties but are rarely mentioned:

CBDA

(Cannabidiolic acid)

Inhibits cancer cell growth

Reduces inflammation

CBC

(Cannabichromene)

Inhibits cancer growth

Stimulates brain growth

Promotes bone growth

Reduces inflammation

Relieves pain

Antibacterial

Antifungal

Anti-depressive

We have established that most of the harmful effects of cannabis on the oral mucosa come from its drying effect, which can lead to tooth decay and gum disease. We have also established that cannabis contains many cannabinoids that are actually beneficial to the oral mucosa, so much so that makers of oral care products are designing products with cannabinoids as the main active ingredients. Smoking cannabis, however, given the comparisons of the carcinogenicity of cannabis smoke to that of tobacco smoke and the former's carcinogenic effects on oral mucosa, will be increasingly challenged as cannabis research reaches full stride.

Although cannabis and tobacco are often casually compared as if the smoke from one is as harmful as the smoke from the other, they are actually quite different in carcinogenic properties. Tobacco contains highly carcinogenic compounds called nitrosamines, which cannabis does not contain. Two of the worst-offending nitrosamines in tobacco are nicotine-derived nitrosamine ketone (NNK) and N-Nitrosonornicotine (NNN) (Hecht and Hoffman 1988).

Dental professionals are in a unique position to offer patient education when it comes to the dry mouth, commonly referred to as "cotton mouth," secondary to smoking cannabis.

When **Neuroprotectant** cannabinoids such as THC bind to CB_1 and CB_2 receptors located in the jaw's submandibular glands, the glands lose their ability to receive input from the parasympathetic nervous system, causing a disruption in normal saliva production.

It's important to take dry mouth seriously, because this "mild" condition is actually anything but. Chronic dry mouth—

technically known as xerostomia, from *xeros*, the Greek word for dry and *stoma* (mouth)—can open the door to a host of negative health effects, including decreased or altered sense of taste; difficulty swallowing and speaking clearly; sore, crusty, cracked skin at the corners of the mouth, which is called angular cheilitis; and the accumulation of dental plaque.

Some plaque buildup is normal and occurs naturally in everyone. However, cannabis users have an increased susceptibility to plaque buildup due to frequent dry mouth. It is important for cannabis users to schedule regular dental cleanings for this reason.

Patient education for cannabis users may include, but not be limited to, the following:

> 1. Keep well hydrated. A general rule of thumb for adequate hydration: divide the patient's weight in half and convert that number to ounces. For example, if a patient weighs one hundred pounds, dividing his or her weight in half gives you fifty pounds. Convert this to fifty ounces, and that would be the amount of a healthy daily intake of water.

> 2. Use sugar-free gum or candy to keep oral mucosa moist.

> 3. Cut down on caffeine intake.

> 4. Try to breathe through the nose instead of the mouth.

> 5. As cannabis causes the "munchies" and dry mouth, always try to brush before sleep.

Chapter 9 References

[1] Cho, C. M., R. Hirsch, and S. Johnstone. 2005. "General and Oral Health Implications of Cannabis Use." *Australian Dental Journal* 50(2): 70–74.
http://www.ncbi.nlm.nih.gov/pubmed/16050084

[2] Hecht, S. S., and Hoffman, D. 1988. "Tobacco-Specific Nitrosamines, an Important Group of Carcinogens in Tobacco and Tobacco Smoke." *Carcinogenesis* 9(6): 875–84.
http://www.ncbi.nlm.nih.gov/pubmed/3286030

[3] Inhale MD. "Is Medical Marijuana Harmful to Dental Health?"
http://inhalemd.com/2015/10/is-medical-marijuana-harmful-to-dental-health/

[4] Nasdaq. 2015. "AXIM Biotechnologies, Inc. Announces Hemp-Based Oral Care Division." February 12.

CHAPTER 10

Cannabis Medicine in Occupational and Physical Therapy

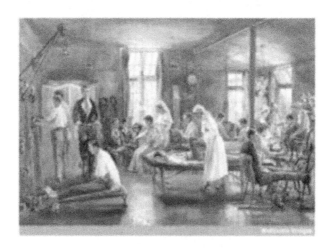

Cannabis Accepted as Medicine

Cannabis has not been universally accepted as a medicine by health care providers in the United States. Veteran hospitals prohibit physicians and patients from discussing and incorporating medical cannabis into the patients' treatment programs. A bipartisan bill was introduced in the US House of Representatives in March of 2016 that would allow the Department of Veterans Affairs physicians to discuss and recommend medical cannabis to their patients in states where medical cannabis is legal.

Due to the ambiguity and disharmony of federal and state laws concerning cannabis, many civilian physicians are hesitant to recommend medical cannabis to their patients out of fear of jeopardy to their licenses. It has been and continues to be a period of great adjustment on the part of health care providers in general.

Medical Cannabis and Pharmaceutical Trends

Regardless of our personal acceptance and belief system around the issue of medical cannabis, the fact remains that we, as health care professionals, now have a responsibility to learn about cannabis as a medicine. Chances are greater than ever before that we will now be working with patients who actively use cannabis as a medicine. If our patients are using it, then we need to know about it. This trend will grow over time. GW Pharmaceuticals, which is located in England, is one of the largest cannabis pharmaceutical companies in the world. Currently, the cannabis-based medications in its development pipeline can be seen below (GW Pharmaceuticals 2014).

GW Pharmaceutical cannabis medication pipeline (R&D)

SATIVEX **CANCER PAIN** (Phase 3 trials ongoing) **MS SPASTICITY** (Phase 3 IND open; SPA-ongoing)
GWP42006 **EPILEPSY** (Phase 2 trial underway)
GWP42003 **NEONATAL HYPOXIC** (Orphan drug designation-received) **ISCHEMIA** **ENCEPHALOPATHY**
GWP42002 **GLIOMA**
GWP42004 **TYPE 2 DIABETES**
GWP42003 **SCHIZOPHRENIA**

New Mexico Medical Cannabis Statistics

As of December 2, 2015

People Seeking Medical Cannabis Relief

(New Mexico Department of Health 2015)

Qualifying Condition Count

Severe chronic pain—6,431

Damage to the nervous tissue of the spinal cord—162

Inflammatory autoimmune-mediated arthritis—342

Spasmodic torticollis (cervical dystonia)—20

Painful peripheral neuropathy—801

Inclusion body myositis—2

Multiple sclerosis—306

Chronic pain—4

Cancer—1,829

Oregon Medical Cannabis Statistics
People Seeking Pain Relief from Medical Cannabis
(Oregon Health Authority 2015)

Receiving medical cannabis for severe pain—67,904

Persistent muscle spasms, including but not limited to epilepsy—20,060

Seizures, including but not limited to epilepsy—1,969

Agitation related to Alzheimer's disease—86

Glaucoma—1,098

HIV/AIDS—732

Cachexia—1,176

Nausea—9,913

Cancer—3,991

PTSD—4,652

The Future Perspective

As highlighted above, 67,904 people in the state of Oregon are legally using medical cannabis for their pain management. That's an astounding figure, would you not agree? As more states get on board and pass medical cannabis laws, these numbers for cannabis pain control will skyrocket, as you would imagine. There will be tens of millions of people in America and around the world using cannabis as a primary medication. This is why it is important to start learning about it now, because before long, we will be seeing it everywhere. When it comes to medicine, this is not recreational; this is full-on cannabis pharmacy.

Balance, cognition, and coordination are all important in the realm of therapy. If people are off balance, they need to be watched. If someone is getting too high, that needs to be assessed. Some botanical strains of medical cannabis can get people very high. In fact, the power and influence of the THC (the psychoactive cannabinoid) can in many cases end up being the limiting factor as to how much cannabis a person can handle. It can be used to treat symptoms successfully, but the ceiling of use is limited by negative tolerance.

Most cannabis users are encouraged to find their own comfort zone of titration. This is often how the prescription for cannabis works. Patients experiment with how much they use, self-assess the effects, and adjust cannabis intake according to what they feel they need. CBD mitigates the THC high.

There are many paradoxes to cannabis therapy that will forever prevent it from fitting in perfectly to the allopathic model of pharmaceutical medications. Although pharmaceutical houses will produce highly regulated cannabis products, the flip side of cannabis therapeutics is that it will always be an ancient, herbal, and botanical medicine and used as such.

The Cost of Cannabis

Cannabinoid medications are expensive and are not covered by insurance. Cannabis is still a Schedule I drug in the United States. Cannabis is classified as the most dangerous of all drugs, having potentially the most severe psychological or physical dependence, and considered to have no acceptable medical use by law; hence insurance companies are not obligated to cover the cost (Good Rx 2016).

1.   **MARINOL**: Approximate cost $200 to $800 per month; $2,400 to $9,600 per year, depending on dosage.

2.   **CESAMET**: Approximate cost $1,150 per month; $13,800 per year.

3.   **SATIVEX**: Approximate cost $1,333 per month; $16,000 per year.

4.   **EPIDIOLEX**: Approximate cost $833 to $1,250 per month; $10,000 to $15,000 per year.

5.   **MEDICAL CANNABIS**: Approximate cost $150 to $400 per ounce; at one ounce per month, $1,800 to $4,800 per year. (Some patients use twice that amount.)

Chapter 10 References

[1] Good Rx. 2016. "Title of Article Needed."
http://www.goodrx.com.
GW Pharmaceuticals. 2014. "Product Pipeline."
http://www.gwpharm.com/product-pipeline.aspx

[2] New Mexico Department of Health. 2015. "Medical Cannabis Program." http://nmhealth.org/publication/view/report/1549/

[3] Oregon Health Authority. 2015. "The Oregon Medical Marijuana Program." .
https://public.health.oregon.gov/DiseasesConditions/ChronicDisease/Me
dicalMarijuanaProgram/Documents/OMMP%20Statistic%20Snapshot%2
0-%2010–2015.pdf/

CHAPTER 11

Pharmacology of Medical Cannabis

Fatal overdose with cannabis alone has not been reported. In terms of acute drug interactions, additive effects of cannabis, anticholinergics, and CNS depressants should be expected (e.g., increased sedation, dizziness, dry mouth, confusion). Cannabinoids are metabolized by several liver enzyme systems, including cytochrome P450 (CYP 2C9, CYP 3A4) and can induce or inhibit CYP 3A4, but there is little evidence of important drug-drug interactions based on CYP 450 systems. Smoking itself (e.g., cannabis or tobacco) induces CYP 1A2 and may increase clearance of some antipsychotics (e.g., olanzapine, clozapine) and antidepressants (e.g., some tricyclics, mirtazepine). Overall then, the acute medical risks of THC as used in clinical trials are rather low. Cannabis will increase the metabolism of theophylline. Research on cannabis-drug interactions is ongoing.

There are risks to be considered in assessing the potential of cannabinoid therapeutics. Cannabis, like other analgesics, can be associated with dependence and a withdrawal syndrome, occurring in a dose-dependent fashion. Under controlled conditions in healthy, experienced users of marijuana, withdrawal from a low daily dose (i.e., oral THC 10 milligrams every 3–4 hours for 5–21 days) commences within twelve hours, is diminished by twenty-four hours, and is complete in forty-eight to seventy-two hours. Other short term experiments with oral THC (20 to 30 milligrams four times daily) and smoked cannabis (1 percent and 3 percent THC cigarettes four times daily) reveal an abstinence syndrome characterized by anxiety, irritability, restlessness, insomnia, stomach pain and, decreased appetite (Grant, Atkinson, Gouaux, and Wilsey 2012).

Entourage Effect

In an article published in *The British Journal of Pharmacology* by Dr. Ethan Russo (Russo 2011), he discusses many, many potential uses for cannabinoid therapy, including anti-inflammatory, analgesic, anticancer, antibiotic, antifungal, anti-nausea, anti-MRSA, antianxiety, memory protection, and reduction of stroke risk.

Although there are synthetic cannabinoid substances produced by pharmaceutical companies, it is believed that the naturally occurring plant substances (phyto-cannabinoids) act synergistically, known as the "entourage effect," for optimal benefits (Leonard-Johnson and Rappaport 2014).

It is this entourage effect that has so many doctors and health professionals convinced that whole plant extracts are more beneficial when taking supplemental cannabinoids.

Side Effects of Cannabis

Adverse side effects of cannabinoids may include the following:

- Low blood pressure
- Rapid beating of the heart
- Muscle relaxation

- Bloodshot eyes

- Slowed digestion

- Dizziness

- Depression

- Hallucinations

- Paranoia

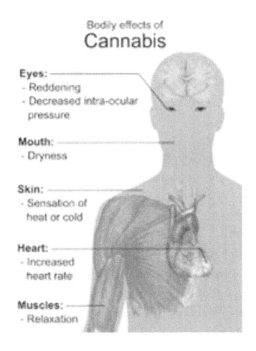

Withdrawal Symptoms from Cannabis

Symptoms of withdrawal from cannabinoids may include the following:

- Trouble sleeping

- Irritability

- Restlessness

- Hot flashes

- Nausea and cramping (These rarely occur.)

Chapter 11 References

[1] Grant, Igor, J., Hampton Atkinson, Ben Gouaux, and Barth Wilsey. 2012. "Medical Marijuana: Clearing Away the Smoke." *Open Neurology Journal* 6: 18–25. http://www.ncbi.nlm.nih.gov/pmc/articles/PMC3358713/.doi: 10.2174/1874205X01206010018

[2] Leonard-Johnson, Steven L., and Tina Rappaport. 2014. *CBD-Rich Hemp Oil: Cannabis Medicine is Back*. Scotts Valley, CA: CreateSpace. https://www.amazon.com/CBD-Rich-Hemp-Oil-Cannabis-Medicine-ebook/dp/B00K8IH3D6?ie=UTF8&qid=1418600126&ref_=tmm_kin_swatch_0&sr=1-1-catcorr

[3] Russo, Ethan. 2011. "Taming THC: Potential Cannabis Synergy and Phytocannabinoid-Terpenoid Entourage Effects." *The British Journal of Pharmacology* Volume, Br J Pharmacol. 2011 Aug; 163(7): 1344–1364. doi: 10.1111/j.1476-5381.2011.01238.x

CHAPTER 12

Routes of Administration and Dosing

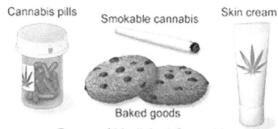

Forms of Medicinal Cannabis

Routes of Administration

1. **VAPORIZING**—Rapid onset within a few minutes, peak onset thirty minutes, and lasts two to four hours. Due to rapid onset, titration is easier to control, especially with inexperienced patients. Vaporizing is just below combustion, thereby reducing the harmful effects of combustion. Vaporizing may be stronger than smoking because less THC is burned off. Requires vaporization equipment and use of vape pens, such as e-cigarettes.

2. **SMOKING**—Rapid onset within a few minutes, avoid smoke form if bronchial irritation present. Smoking cannabis will have varied titration.

3. **INGESTING**—Baked goods, extracted powder, or tinctures. Less predictable, longer effect (up to five to eight hours). Thirty minutes to two hours onset, best for experienced users, may use for pain protection for a night.

4.   **SUBLINGUAL**—Tincture by eye dropper under the tongue.

5.   **TOPICAL**—Pharmokinetics not clear, no psychoactive effects when applied topically, many anecdotal success stories.

6.   **RECTAL**—Less common. However, absorption rate superior to ingested cannabis.

7.   **VAGINAL**—The newest type of cannabis delivery system used for conditions such as menstrual pain and vaginal inflammation.

8.   **EYE DROPS**—For treatment of glaucoma.

As little as 2.5 milligrams of THC may have a clinical therapeutic value. This amount is generally considered a starting dose until the patient gains experience with taking cannabis and gets familiar with the effects of cannabis on him or her. A patient learns to titrate his or her own dosage needs over time. Follow-up visits are important after initiating cannabis treatment in order to assess the patient for any difficulties he or she may be experiencing with the treatment.

In the case of smoked/vaporized cannabis, the dose required to achieve therapeutic effects and avoid adverse effects is difficult to estimate and is affected by the source of the plant material, its processing and different smoking techniques. These techniques include depth of inhalation, duration of breath holding, and the number and frequency of puffs, as well as how much of the cigarette is smoked or how much plant material is vaporized. Smoking or vaporization should proceed slowly and cautiously in a gradual fashion and should cease if the patient begins to experience the following effects: disorientation, dizziness, ataxia, agitation, anxiety, tachycardia and orthostatic hypotension, depression, hallucinations, or psychosis (Health Canada 2013).

There is also insufficient information regarding oral dosing, but the patient should be made aware that the effects following oral administration only begin to be felt thirty minutes to an hour or more after ingestion, that consumption of cannabis-based products (e.g., cookies, baked goods) should proceed slowly, and that edibles should be consumed only in small amounts at a time in order to gauge the effects and to prevent overdosing.

It is always recommended that a patient start off with low dose and go slowly when initiating cannabis treatment. A follow-up visit can be done within a few weeks to assess how well the patient is doing and to see if any modifications to the treatment are needed. The patient should be encouraged to keep a cannabis journal. In the journal, information such as time cannabis was taken, how much was consumed, any side effects, pain relief, and general tolerance to cannabis therapy should be entered. A journal will show a pattern of use the physician will use to make further assessments. Assessment will include how to titrate other medications being taken, if needed, after initiating cannabis therapy.

In a case in which it is indicated that cannabis therapy should be discontinued, it is recommended that a 20 percent decrease in cannabis consumption daily be initiated in order to minimize withdrawal from cannabis. Withdrawal symptoms may include anxiety, irritability, restlessness, insomnia, stomach pain, and a decreased appetite.

Chapter 12 References

[1] Health Canada. 2013-06-12 . "Information for Health Care Professionals."
http://www.hc-sc.gc.ca/dhp-mps/marihuana/med/infoprof-eng.php

CHAPTER 13

Contraindications to Cannabinoid Therapy

I would like to start off by saying that nothing is written in stone when it comes to cannabis. Research is coming down the pipeline fast and furious. Some of what we thought were potential harmful effects of cannabis are now being disproven: for instance, that cannabis is harmful to the lungs. This theory is now being challenged, along with many other theories about the negative effects of cannabis. Listed below are the current contraindications, and these are subject to change at any time, based on research as it evolves.

The contraindications that apply to those considering using prescription cannabinoid-based therapies (such as nabilone [Cesamet], nabiximols [Sativex], or dronabinol [Marinol]) also apply to those considering using whole-plant cannabis. Side effects of cannabinoid extracts and synthetics may be more severe in nature.

Currently, no clinical guidelines exist with respect to monitoring patients who are taking cannabis for therapeutic purposes. The risk-benefit ratio of using cannabis should be carefully evaluated in patients with the following medical conditions because of individual variation in response and tolerance to its effects, as well as the difficulty in dosing (Health Canada 2013):

1.   Cannabis should be used cautiously with any person under the age of eighteen and in any patient who has a history of hypersensitivity to any cannabinoid or to smoke. The adverse effects of cannabis use on mental

health are greater during development, particularly during adolescence, than in adulthood. (Epidiolex is THC-free and is used for seizures in children.)

2.   Cannabis should be used with caution in patients with a history of substance abuse, including alcohol abuse, because such individuals may be more prone to abuse cannabis, which itself is a frequently abused substance. Substance-abuse screening tools may be used to assess patients with a history of substance abuse.

3.   Cannabis should not be used in patients with severe liver or renal disease. Patients with ongoing chronic hepatitis C should be strongly advised to abstain from daily cannabis use, as this has been shown to be a predictor of steatosis severity in these individuals.

4.   Cannabis should not be used in patients with a personal history of psychiatric disorders (especially schizophrenia) or a familial history of schizophrenia. (More studies are needed to assess cannabis's true effect on schizophrenia. There are studies currently underway to see if there are any benefits cannabis has on schizophrenia, PTSD, anxiety, depression, and ADHD.) As previously mentioned, old belief systems about cannabis are currently being challenged and shattered, and in some cases, and as studies progress, the real story on the therapeutic benefits of cannabis will be revealed.

5.   Cannabis should not be used in patients with severe cardiopulmonary disease, because of occasional

hypotension, possible hypertension, syncope, or tachycardia.

6.   Smoked cannabis is not recommended in patients with respiratory insufficiency, such as asthma or chronic obstructive pulmonary disease.

7.   Patients with mania or depression and using cannabis or a cannabinoid should be under careful psychiatric monitoring. Cannabis should be used with caution in patients receiving concomitant therapy with sedative-resistive or psychoactive effects.

8.   Cannabis may also exacerbate the CNS depressant effects of alcohol and increase the incidence of adverse effects.

9.   Patients should be advised of the negative effects of cannabis/cannabinoids on memory and to report any mental or behavioral changes that occur after using cannabis. (needs more studies)

Cannabis is not recommended in women of childbearing age who are not on a reliable contraceptive or those planning pregnancy, those who are pregnant, or women who are breastfeeding. (Again, this concept is being challenged and needs more studies.)

Pros of Cannabis as a Medicine

- Has a very good risk vs. value profile.

- Has low abuse potential (equal to caffeine).

- No one has ever fatally overdosed using medical cannabis.

- Plant-based cannabis is better tolerated than synthetic THC medications.

- Has a broad spectrum of benefits when introduced in the endocannabinoid system.

- Side-effect/adverse-effect profiles are mild to moderate.

- Does not suppress respiratory function.

Cons of Cannabis as a Medicine

- Reduced balance and coordination.

- Impairment of thinking, problem-solving skills, and memory.

- Potential for hallucinations and withdrawal symptoms.

- Long-term users may need higher doses. May be an indication for a medication holiday.

- Lowered reaction times and altered perception.

- Not covered by insurance; patient/family will have to pay for it out of pocket.

- Tolerance may develop.

• Studies have been inhibited due to Schedule I status. (More studies are needed.)

• Has street value, but not as much as opioids.

Chapter 13 References

[1] Health Canada. 2013-06-12. "Information for Health Care Professionals."
http://www.hc-sc.gc.ca/dhp-mps/marihuana/med/infoprof-eng.php

CHAPTER 14

Patient and Family Education

1. Cannabis may not work for everyone; however, cannabis has been a useful tool in helping reduce pain and increase function.

2. Not all cannabis strains are created equally; some strains may work to relieve pain, and others may not be as effective. Cannabis strain is important, so the patient may need to try different types before reaching success.

3. It is important to eat edibles slowly—perhaps one bite every thirty to sixty minutes. The effects come on slowly, and it is easy to consume more than needed when effects are slow in coming.

4. Many health providers are still uncomfortable recommending medical cannabis due to inconsistencies in federal and state laws. Also, the variety of cannabis strains can make it challenging for a provider to predict what the effect might be.

5. Contraindications are suggested; however, the patient and the health care provider can do a risk versus benefit analysis, and appropriateness of cannabis use, route, and dosage can be determined. As more studies are conducted, the risk profiles of medical cannabis are constantly being reevaluated, and changing. This also includes people with a history of addiction, as cannabis is now being viewed as a therapeutic medicine for opioid addiction. The state of

Maine is now considering adding cannabis as a therapy for opioid addiction and as a qualifying diagnosis to receive a medical cannabis recommendation.

6. Cannabis medications with a one-to-one THC-to-CBD ratio, such as Sativex, have a very safe record. Sativex has mild side effects, is low in adverse effects, and tends to have a milder withdrawal than high THC, low CBD strains of cannabis. The most common side effects of Sativex are fatigue and dizziness. Sativex has not produced any mental health or cognition problems, as can happen with the higher THC strains.

7. Cannabis side effects are mild compared to those of opioid medication.

8. Cannabis can have a synergistic effect with opioid medications.

9. Cannabis can decrease pain in some people without increasing their opioid medication. In some instances, cannabis used with opioid medications can lower the opioid dosage with the same analgesic effect as using a higher dose of an opioid medication alone. Cannabis may surpass the effects of an opioid medication and be used as a stand-alone medication.

10. Patients should be encouraged to speak with their providers about the best delivery system of cannabis to achieve the most relief with the least number of side effects. Consider also that some routes of administration are more expensive and may be more or less therapeutic.

11. Reassure the patient and his/her family members that, as he or she gains experience with using cannabis, starting low and going slow, he or she will get better at the art of using cannabis as a medication.

12. Teach that the desired outcome is symptom relief, not getting high. The goal is to get the most relief with the least amount of intoxication or completely without intoxication.

13. A provider can recommend dosing; however, fundamentally, cannabis is self-titrated to some degree. Reassure patients that if they take too much cannabis, adverse effects will gradually subside. Edibles have the highest risk of the patient getting too much, so if a patient is taking edibles, he or she must go very low and slow, especially at the start of treatment.

14. Patients should notify their providers if they have adverse effects.

15. Some patients may want to keep journals of their experiences with different strains, the amounts taken, and the effects and relief experienced. A journal can also help the provider make an accurate assessment of cannabis treatment (risk versus benefit analysis).

16. Discuss possible impairment using cannabis, and caution patient not to drive or operate equipment.

17. Encourage follow-up visits. This is especially important when the patient is taking other medications, to evaluate the titration of all medications, their effectiveness, and any issues that may come up during cannabis treatment.

About the Author

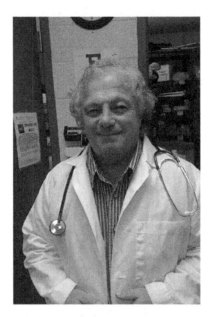

Steven Leonard-Johnson
RN-BC, PhD, LMT, BCB

Steven is a current member of the American Cannabis Nurses Association (ACNA).

He is certified as a Psychiatric and Mental Health Nurse by the American Nurses Credentialing Center. Steve has many years of experience working in the acute care psychiatric setting including the emergency room, geriatric, forensic, acute detox, adult, dual diagnosis and intensive care psychiatric units. Steve has worked in New York metropolitan area hospitals and spent five years in home health care as a psychiatric nurse in an under-served, rural area of Maine.

Steve is also a Senior Fellow with the Biofeedback Certification International Alliance. Certified by the National Certification Board for Therapeutic Massage and Bodywork, Steve is an active member of the American Massage Therapy Association. His area of clinical interest is in the study of mind/body interaction preferring holistic treatment of pain, anxiety and trauma; he has developed a sophisticated style in deep tissue massage using CBD oil, infrared heat and high speed vibration as the base and he is writing about it in his next book, using his many years as a medical massage therapist as his guide.

Steve is an active member of American Mensa and Intertel societies.

Steve is coauthor of *CBD-Rich Hemp Oil: Cannabis Medicine Is Back*, a number-one Amazon best seller in eleven countries in the category of psychopharmacology.

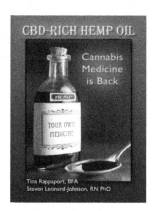

About the Editor

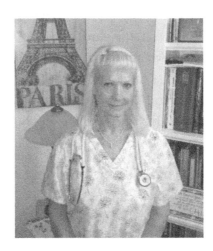

Kelly F. Walker
RN-BC, PhD, NCSN

Kelly has been a dedicated nurse for more than thirty years. Kelly is a nurse's nurse: an excellent pediatric and adolescent psychiatric nurse. She has been certified in psychiatric and mental health nursing by the American Nurses Credentialing Center. She is also certified by the National Board for Certification of School Nurses in school nursing.

Kelly has served as a director of nursing at an ICF/MR intermediate care facility for individuals with mental retardation (ICF/MR). She has years of experience working in acute care, dual diagnosis, forensics, and child and adolescent residential psychiatry. Kelly has also worked for many years in a school health setting.

Her area of clinical interest is acute care psychiatric nursing, with a specialization in the care and treatment of children and adolescents. Kelly's dissertation title was "Substance Abuse Treatment in Health Care Professionals." It was an eye-opening study on a topic that is not often discussed.

She has practiced in southeast Florida and in the Catskills area of New York, where she grew up.

Five Continuing Education Credits for

Health Care Professionals

If you are interested in professional, accredited CEU's, please follow this link to a cannabis related course I developed for the following professions

Coursework was designed primarily for, but not limited to, the following professional categories:

- Nurses

- Dentists

- Physical therapists

- Physical therapy assistants

- Occupational therapists

- Pharmacists

The course has been completed and is now available online. It is for 5 CEUs and is approved in all states by most of the state boards for the professions mentioned above.

5 CEUs on this topic, click the link below. The cost of the course is $40.00.

http://blxtraining.com/Medical%20Cannabis%20in%20Pain%20Management.pdf

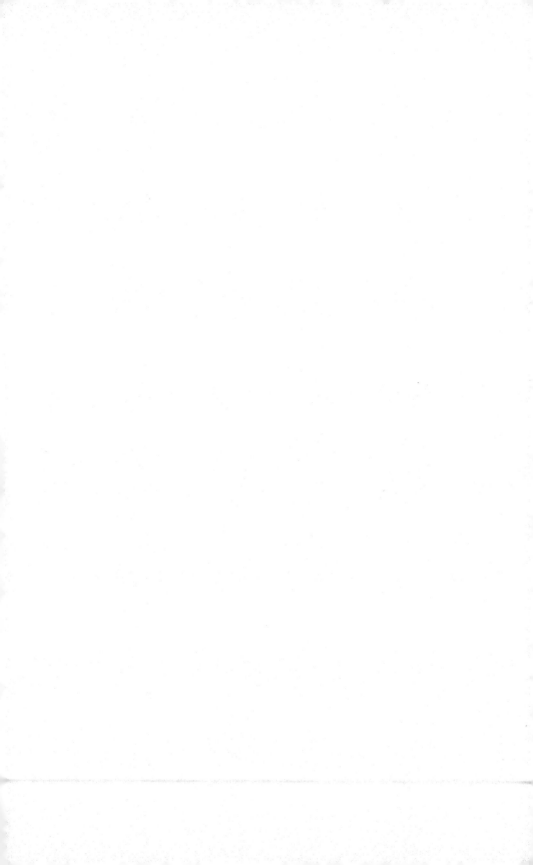

Made in the USA
Monee, IL
30 August 2020